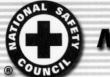 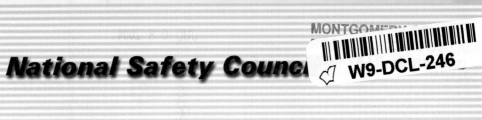
National Safety Council

Pediatric
First Aid and CPR

Fourth Edition

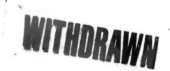

JONES AND BARTLETT PUBLISHERS
Sudbury, Massachusetts
BOSTON   TORONTO   LONDON   SINGAPORE

Jones and Bartlett Publishers
40 Tall Pine Drive, Sudbury, MA 01776
978-443-5000
nsc@jbpub.com
Internet: http://www.nsc.jbpub.com/nsc/

Jones and Bartlett Publishers Canada
2406 Nikanna Road
Mississauga, ON L5C 2W6
CANADA

Jones and Bartlett Publishers International
Barb House, Barb Mews
London W6 7PA
UK

 National Safety Council ®
First Aid Institute
1121 Spring Lake Drive
Itasca, IL 60143-3201
(630) 285-1121
(800) 621-7619
www.nsc.org

*Executive Director, Home & Community
Safety and Health Group:* Donna Siegfried

*Program Development & Training Manager,
Home & Community Safety and Health
Group:* Barbara Caracci

Copyright © 2001 by Jones and Bartlett Publishers, Inc.

The first aid and CPR procedures in this book are based on the most current recommendations of responsible medical sources. The National Safety Council and the publisher, however, make no guarantee as to, and assume no responsibility for, the correctness, sufficiency or completeness of such information or recommendations. Other or additional safety measures may be required under particular circumstances.

Library of Congress Cataloging-in-Publication Data
First Aid and CPR, standard / National Safety Council.—4th ed.
    p.   cm.
    Includes index.
    ISBN 0-7637-1322-8
    1. Pediatric emergencies.   2. First aid in illness and injury.   3. CPR (First aid) for children.   4. CPR (First aid) for infants.   I. National Safety Council.
    RJ370.P4575 2001
    616.92'0025–dc21

2001029414

Chief Executive Officer: Clayton E. Jones
Chief Operating Officer: Donald W. Jones, Jr.
Executive V.P. and Publisher: Tom Manning
V.P. and Managing Editor: Judith H. Hauck
V.P., Production and Design: Anne Spencer
*V.P., Manufacturing and
    Inventory Control:* Therese Bräuer
Publisher, EMS & Aquatics: Lawrence D. Newell
Emergency Care Acquisitions Editor: Kimberly Brophy
Emergency Care Associate Editor: Jennifer Reed
Production Editors: Cynthia J. Korisky, Jennifer Angel
Writers: Stephanie O'Neill, Connie Page, Alton Thygerson
Text Design: Studio Montage
Illustrations: Rolin Graphics
Cover Design: Studio Montage
Cover Photographs (clockwise from top left):
    © Brian Pieters/Materfile;
    AFP/Corbis;
    Steve Ferry/P&F Communications;
    Jones and Bartlett Publishers
Printing and Binding: Courier Company

Interior Stock Photos:
    Chapter 1: Opener © Bronwyn Kidd/Photodisc;
    Figure 1 Courtesy of the American Academy of Pediatrics
    Chapter 2: Opener © Linda Gheen
    Chapter 3: Opener © Lincoln Russell/PictureQuest
    Chapter 4: Opener © IT Stock International
    Chapter 5: Opener © Steve Perry/P&P Communications
    Chapter 6: Opener © William Johnson/PictureQuest
    Chapter 7: Opener © Stephen Agricola/PictureQuest
    Chapter 8: Opener © Russell Illig/Photodisc
    Chapter 9: Opener © Stephen Agricola/PictureQuest
    Chapter 10: Opener © David Dennis/Animals Animals;
    Figure 1 © 1998 Jim Markham; **Figure 2** © 1995 Wedgworth/ Custom Medical Stock Photo; **Figure 3** © S.J. Krasemann/Peter Arnold, Inc.; **Figure 7** © 1998 Lance Beeny
    Chapter 11: Opener © 1998, Dave Lissy/Index Stock Photography
    Chapter 12: Opener © Richard Wool/Index Stock Photography, 1998
    Chapter 13: Opener © Keith/Custom Medical Stock Photo
    Chapter 14: Opener © Richard Radstone
    Chapter 15: Opener 2001 James Darrell/Stone Images
    Chapter 16: Opener and Figure 4 © Bob Daemmrich/ PictureQuest; **Figure 3** © O.J. Staats/Custom Medical Stock Photo; **Figures 6 and 7** © NMSB/Custom Medical Stock Photo; **Figure 8** © Dr. H.C. Robinson/Science Photo Library; **Figure 10** © Science Photo Library

Printed in the United States of America
04 03 02   10 9 8 7 6 5 4 3

About the National Safety Council Program

Congratulations on selecting the National Safety Council's First Aid and CPR program! You join good company, as the National Safety Council has successfully trained over 6 million people worldwide in first aid and cardiopulmonary resuscitation (CPR). The National Safety Council's training network of nearly 10,000 instructors at over 4,000 sites worldwide has established the National Safety Council programs as the standard by which all others are judged.

In setting the standards, the National Safety Council has worked in close cooperation with hundreds of national and international organizations, thousands of corporations, thousands of leading educators, dozens of leading medical organizations, and hundreds of state and local governmental agencies. Their collective input has helped create programs that stand alone in quality. Consider just a few of the National Safety Council's current collaborations:

World's Leading Medical Organizations

The National Safety Council is currently working with both the American Academy of Orthopedic Surgeons (AAOS), Wilderness Medical Society (WMS), and the American Heart Association to help bring innovative, new training programs to the marketplace. The National Safety Council and the AAOS are developing a new First Responder program and the National Safety Council and the WMS are developing the first-of-its-kind wilderness first aid program.

Spanning the Globe

Across the globe, from Boston to Bangkok, from Miami to Milan, from Seattle to Stockholm, people are trained with National Safety Council programs. National Safety Council first aid and CPR programs are already used in your area.

World's Leading Corporations

Thousands of corporations including Westinghouse, Exxon, General Motors, Pacific Bell, Ameritech, and U.S. West have selected many of the National Safety Council emergency care programs to train employees.

World's Leading Colleges and Universities

Hundreds of leading colleges and universities are working closely with the National Safety Council to fully develop and implement the Internet Initiative that will establish the National Safety Council as the leading online provider of emergency care programs.

Most importantly, in selecting the National Safety Council programs, you can feel confident that the programs are accepted and approved worldwide. You can rely on the National Safety Council. Founded in 1913, the National Safety Council is dedicated to protecting life, promoting health, and reducing accidental death. For more than 80 years, the National Safety Council has been the world's leading authority on safety/injury education.

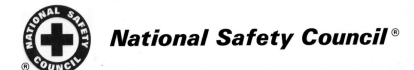

Table of Contents

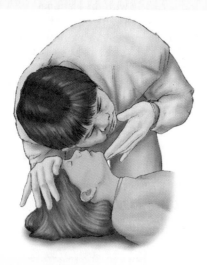

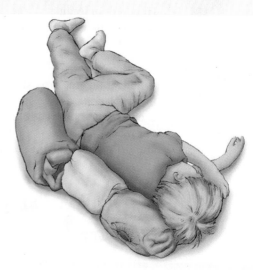

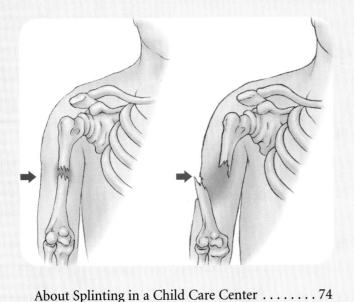

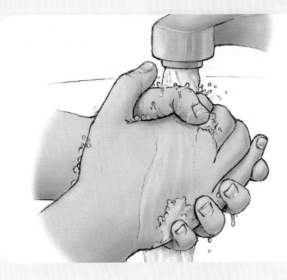

Your First Aid & CPR IQ

Test your current knowledge. Read each question and place your answer in the "Pre-check" column. After reading this manual and completing your course, read the questions again and place your answers in the "Post-check" column. Compare your answers and see what you have learned.

Question	Pre-check			Post-check		
1. Poisoning is the number one cause of death in children.	T	F	Uncertain	T	F	Uncertain
2. Hives are a sign of an allergic reaction.	T	F	Uncertain	T	F	Uncertain
3. Butter on a burn helps to reduce pain.	T	F	Uncertain	T	F	Uncertain
4. Bleeding from veins spurts and is difficult to control.	T	F	Uncertain	T	F	Uncertain
5. Rabies is passed in the saliva of animals.	T	F	Uncertain	T	F	Uncertain
6. Heat stroke can be life-threatening.	T	F	Uncertain	T	F	Uncertain
7. The scrubbing motion is just as important as using soap when washing hands.	T	F	Uncertain	T	F	Uncertain
8. Syrup of ipecac causes vomiting.	T	F	Uncertain	T	F	Uncertain
9. First aid for a burn includes applying ice.	T	F	Uncertain	T	F	Uncertain
10. Gloves keep fingers warmer than mittens.	T	F	Uncertain	T	F	Uncertain
11. Shivering increases the body's temperature.	T	F	Uncertain	T	F	Uncertain
12. Frostbitten toes should be rewarmed with gentle massage.	T	F	Uncertain	T	F	Uncertain
13. A child with heat exhaustion has a normal body temperature.	T	F	Uncertain	T	F	Uncertain
14. A child experiencing anaphylaxis needs sugar immediately.	T	F	Uncertain	T	F	Uncertain
15. A bite that breaks the skin can become infected.	T	F	Uncertain	T	F	Uncertain
16. One dose of tetanus vaccine provides immunization for a life-time.	T	F	Uncertain	T	F	Uncertain
17. A wound can be sutured up to 24 hours after the injury.	T	F	Uncertain	T	F	Uncertain
18. The sun's rays are the strongest between 2 p.m. and 4 p.m.	T	F	Uncertain	T	F	Uncertain
19. The reflection of the sun off water or sand increases the intensity.	T	F	Uncertain	T	F	Uncertain
20. Pain medication should not be given to a child with a head injury.	T	F	Uncertain	T	F	Uncertain
21. To stop a nosebleed, place pressure on the upper lip.	T	F	Uncertain	T	F	Uncertain
22. First aid for a bone, joint, or muscle injury includes applying heat to reduce swelling.	T	F	Uncertain	T	F	Uncertain
23. The recovery position helps to prevent a child from choking.	T	F	Uncertain	T	F	Uncertain
24. Poison ivy spreads from contact with open blisters.	T	F	Uncertain	T	F	Uncertain
25. Children most commonly choke on small toy pieces.	T	F	Uncertain	T	F	Uncertain

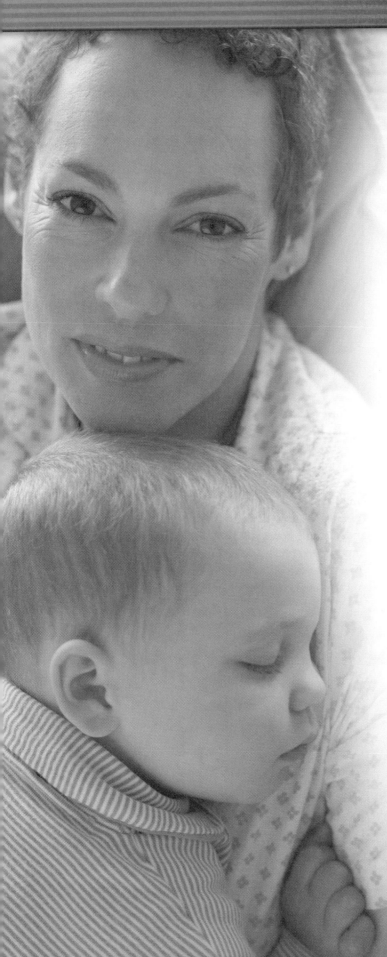

Chapter 1

Background Information

Before You Begin

It is indeed wonderful to be greeted by a young child's smile and a hug or to be shown a special piece of artwork by its proud creator, and there are few experiences warmer than holding a child on your lap while you read a favorite story. Despite the runny noses, diapers, spilled milk, and other, less attractive tasks that are part of your day, the emotional rewards of child care are tremendously satisfying.

As a child care provider, you have the important job of caring for and nurturing young children. In addition to the nurturing aspects of your work, you must be thinking constantly about the safety of children. Ordinary adult habits—such as leaving a purse on the floor, setting a pair of scissors on the counter, placing a cup of hot coffee on the kitchen table, keeping vitamins at the bathroom sink, or leaving a second-story window open—present potentially dangerous situations for children. The protective environment you create and your influence and example help to guide children safely in their development toward becoming creative, self-assured, and considerate people.

Preventing Childhood Injuries

In the United States, unintentional injuries are the leading health problem for children 1 to 16 years of age. According to the National Safety Council, injuries cause more deaths among children than all diseases combined and are the leading cause of disability. Each year, an estimated 600,000 children are hospitalized for injuries, and almost 16 million are seen in emergency medical facilities for treatment.

The Center for Disease Control estimates that more than 30,000 children suffer permanent disabilities from injuries each year. These disabilities have enormous adverse effects on a child's development and future productivity and severely strain the financial and emotional resources of families.

Unintentional injuries are often referred to as accidents because they occur unexpectedly and seem uncontrollable. But most accidents are better termed "preventable" injuries. They can be avoided if a few simple injury-prevention steps are practiced consistently. Unfortunately, injuries occur if these steps are ignored.

Consider the injury that results when a young child swallows a cleaning product that was not properly stored or when a toddler falls down a flight of stairs that did not have a stairway gate in place. Such preventable injuries threaten the health and safety of children who cannot yet protect themselves and leave the adult filled with worry and regrets.

Public education and awareness programs can and do reduce the numbers of childhood injuries and deaths. Thousands more could be avoided every year through currently available prevention strategies. For example:

- The enforcement of state seat belt laws and child safety restraint laws, plus the efforts to reduce drunk driving, help reduce vehicle-related injuries and deaths (▶ Figure 1-1).

- Public awareness and use of smoke detectors has reduced injuries and deaths from home fires.

- Product safety testing on juvenile products has significantly reduced injuries to young children.

- The proper use of bicycle helmets has reduced the number and severity of head injuries.

- Educational programs for preschool and elementary school children on fire prevention, poison prevention, motor vehicle restraints, and water safety have all helped decrease the number of these injuries to children (▼ Figure 1-2).

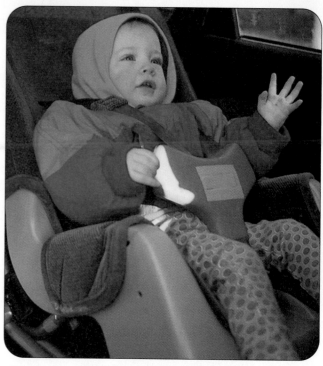

Figure 1-1   Child safety seat.

However, even the best injury-prevention strategies cannot prevent all mishaps. When a child's bicycle tire hits a rock and the child falls, skinning an elbow or breaking an arm, it is still, and always will be, an unpreventable incident that is part of the passage through childhood.

Being aware of the dangers in a child's environment and knowing how you can make that environment safer are important in preventing childhood injuries (▼ Figure 1-3). Injury prevention steps can reduce the likelihood that you will need to use your first aid skills.

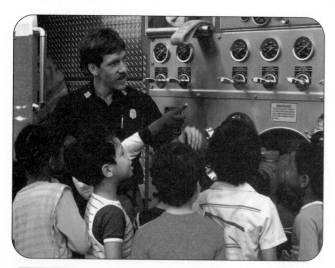

Figure 1-2   Use advocacy to help prevent injuries.

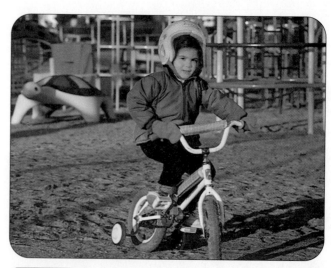

Figure 1-3   Wearing a helmet can prevent serious injuries.

Importance of First Aid

First aid is the immediate care given to an injured or suddenly ill person. It provides temporary assistance until medical care, if needed, is obtained. In fact, most injuries and sudden illnesses require no more than first aid care. However, proper first aid can also mean the difference between life and death, rapid and slow recovery, or temporary and permanent disability.

Injuries can occur no matter how caring or watchful adults are and despite the best safety plans. Because of the frequency of injuries to children, it is likely that a child care provider will be present when an injury or sudden illness occurs. The types of injuries that occur often directly relate to the child's age and developmental level. (See *Common Injuries Related to Child's Developmental Level* in Chapter 17.) Planning to prevent these injuries is essential, and it is equally essential to master first aid techniques.

Legal Aspects of First Aid

No one is required to provide first aid unless a legal obligation to do so exists. Moral obligations may exist, but they are not the same as legal obligations.

A person has a legal responsibility to act in the following situations:

- When employment requires it. The responsibility for the safety of other people is inherent in some jobs, such as police officer, lifeguard, chauffeur, teacher, and child care provider.

- When a pre-existing relationship exists. When there is a pre-existing relationship between two people, such as between a parent and a child or between an adult driver and a child rider in the vehicle, the adult has a responsibility to provide or to obtain first aid care, if necessary.

In addition, once a person begins treating a child for an injury, the care giver must not stop until relieved by another competent adult, until emergency medical help arrives, or until the care giver is physically exhausted.

First Aid Training

Delivering high quality first aid care is necessary, and maintaining standards in the training of first aiders is essential. The National Safety Council first aid and cardiopulmonary resuscitation (CPR) programs meet the requirements of state regulations and follow the latest first aid and CPR procedures established by national emergency care and safety-related organizations. A trained first aider should provide appropriate care only within the scope of the training he or she has received.

Permission and First Aid

A person should always obtain permission before giving first aid. Most child care centers require parents to complete forms giving their permission to have the child treated in an emergency.

If you don't know the injured child, you must first obtain permission to deliver first aid from the parent or guardian. Verbal consent is acceptable. Tell the parent that you are trained in first aid and explain what you plan to do. If a parent or guardian is not available, emergency lifesaving first aid may be given without consent, because it is assumed that the child's parent(s) would consent in this instance.

Combative older children who threaten to harm themselves or others can present difficult management problems. Remember that, although infrequently needed, police officers have the authority to restrain and transport a child as well as an adult.

Rarely, a first aider encounters a parent who refuses to give permission. When this occurs, it is usually done on the basis of moral, ethical, or religious grounds. Call for emergency medical help and allow professionals to deal with the situation.

Good Samaritan Laws

In most emergencies, you are not legally required to give first aid. To encourage people to assist others who need help, Good Samaritan laws grant immunity against lawsuits. Although laws vary from state to state, Good Samaritan immunity generally applies only when the rescuer is: (1) acting during an emergency, (2) acting in good faith, which means he or she has good intentions, (3) acting without compensation, and (4) not guilty of any malicious misconduct or gross negligence toward the victim.

Good Samaritan laws are not a substitute for competent first aid or for keeping within the scope of your training. To find out about your state's Good Samaritan laws, ask for information at your local library.

Disease Precautions

Most people are aware that serious illnesses can be passed from one person to another. They may hesitate to risk their own health for the sake of a stranger. It is only normal to have these worries.

Knowing how germs are transmitted and how to protect yourself from disease while giving first aid enables you to act wisely and with confidence.

Take Steps Now...

1. Post emergency numbers, including the poison control center, next to every telephone.

2. Keep a well-stocked first aid kit in your center and one for travel. Routinely check and replace products that have been used or have expired.

3. Be sure all staff members know first aid and CPR. Check your state's requirements by contacting your state's licensing agency.

4. Have disposable gloves available.

5. Be sure your center's name and building address are clearly posted outside.

6. Check the batteries in smoke detectors in the spring and fall when you change your clocks.

7. Make sure your center has a fire escape plan, including a meeting spot outside. Practice this plan with the children.

8. Know the location of your fire extinguisher. Do not store it near a stove or other location where a fire might prevent you from reaching it when you need to use it.

9. Always use seat belts. Ask parents to transport children in age-appropriate child safety restraints.

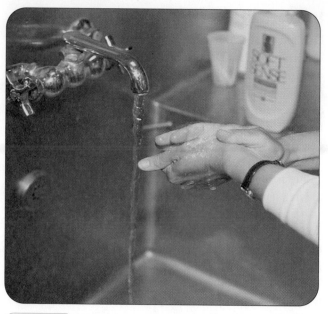

Figure 1-4   Illustration of handwashing.

Germs are everywhere—in homes, work places, and schools—wherever people gather together. And when people are together, the spread of illness is to be expected. The best known illness-causing germs, or microorganisms, are bacteria and viruses. Although not all bacteria and viruses cause illness, a small number do and some of them can be deadly.

Infections caused by bacteria, such as strep throat and many ear infections, are treated with antibiotics. Infections caused by viruses, such as the common cold, have no specific medicines to cure them. There are medicines to relieve unpleasant symptoms of a viral infection, but the body must rely on its immune system to destroy a virus. Unfortunately, a few viruses cannot be subdued by the immune system and can destroy it, threatening the life of the individual. The human immunodeficiency virus (HIV), which causes AIDS, and the hepatitis B and C viruses behave in this way.

Organisms that cause disease enter the body in 1 of 4 ways: touch, ingestion, inhalation, and blood-to-blood exchange. When giving first aid care, you can reduce your risk of contracting or transmitting disease by following these guidelines:

- Wear disposable gloves when giving first aid.

- If disposable gloves are not available, use another barrier, such as a thickly-folded towel, a plastic bag, or several thick layers of gauze pads. Plastic wrap placed over the gauze or towel increases the effectiveness of the barrier.

- Wash your hands immediately after removing disposable gloves. Use antimicrobial wipes if hand-washing facilities are unavailable ▲ Figure 1-4 .

Caution:

DO NOT touch blood, other body fluids, or fluid-tinged clothing with ungloved hands.

DO NOT eat, drink, or touch your face while giving first aid.

First Aid Supplies

Although you hope an emergency never occurs, you need to be prepared. Part of being prepared means keeping a well-stocked first aid kit. You will be better able to act efficiently in an emergency if you have the necessary supplies on hand.

Store all supplies in a locked container out of the reach of children. Plastic tool or tackle boxes make good containers for first aid supplies because they are lightweight, sturdy, and portable, and close securely. Keep the container in a cool, dry location. Make sure every staff member knows where the kit is stored. Remember to take your traveling first aid kit along on a field trip.

Antibiotics and other medicines prescribed for a child's illness should not be stored in the first aid kit. Many of these medicines must be refrigerated. Check the first aid kit regularly for items that have been used and replace them. Discard expired items.

Supplies for a first aid kit include:

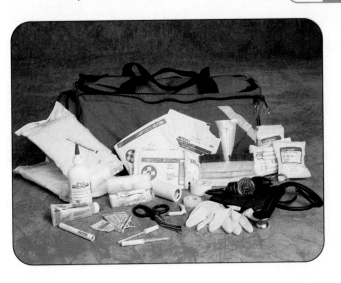

- Adhesive bandages (assorted sizes)
- CPR mouth barriers (child and infant sizes)
- Commercial cold pack
- Cotton swabs
- Disposable gloves
- Eye pads
- Gauze pads (assorted sizes)
- Measuring spoons
- Nonstick sterile pads (assorted sizes)
- Rolled elastic bandages (assorted sizes)
- Rolled gauze bandages (assorted sizes)
- Syrup of ipecac
- Scissors
- Sling or triangular bandages
- Tape (adhesive or other first aid types)
- Thermometer (digital)
- Tongue depressor
- Tweezers
- White cotton handkerchief

In addition, you might want to include the items below. Know your center's policies regarding the use of these products.

- Acetaminophen
- Baking soda
- Calamine lotion
- Oil of cloves
- Topical antibiotic ointments

An emergency kit for use with severe allergic reactions (also known as an insect sting kit), if prescribed by a physician for a specific child in your center, should be kept with the first aid supplies.

Learning Activities

Before You Begin

Directions: Circle Yes if you agree with the statement, and circle No if you disagree.

(Yes) No **1.** A first aider can reduce the risk of transmitting disease by wearing disposable gloves when giving first aid.

Yes (No) **2.** Most injuries and sudden illnesses require no more than first aid care.

Yes (No) **3.** The types of injuries that occur to children often relate to their age and developmental level.

Yes (No) **4.** First aiders can attempt to provide emergency first aid care beyond their scope of training if they feel it would help the injured person.

(Yes) No **5.** Child care providers have a legal obligation to provide first aid to children in their care.

(Yes) No **6.** Written or verbal permission must be obtained before a first aider can give emergency life-saving care.

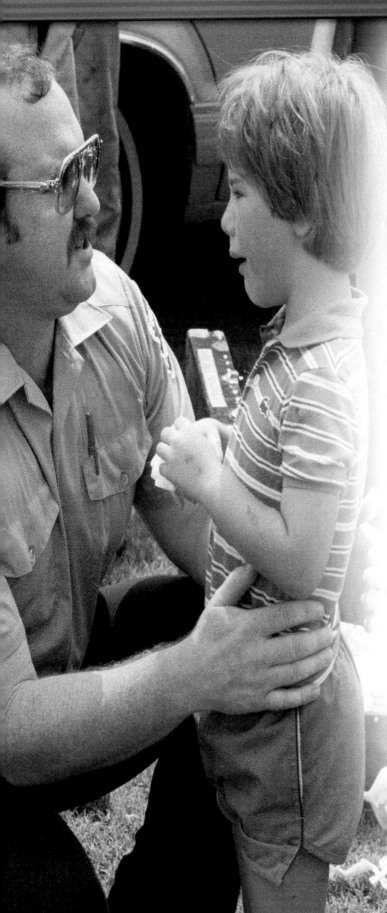

Chapter 2

Finding Out What's Wrong

Handling an Emergency

During an emergency that involves a child, it is essential for you to remain calm and in control. Your calm attitude and methodical approach will inspire the confidence of an injured child and set a standard for other adults to follow.

Your actions in giving first aid should never contribute to making a condition worse. Always handle an injured or ill child gently and avoid any unnecessary movements that might aggravate the problem.

Scene Survey

When an injury or illness occurs, take a moment to figure out what might have happened and how to proceed. Check the scene for:

- Safety
- Clues
- Number of victims

Check the scene to make sure that it is safe for you to approach. In most childhood injury situations, there will be no hazards to your safety. However, if there are, do not risk making yourself another victim. For instance, be alert for unusual dangers, such as deep water, downed electrical wires, or chemical fumes. Before you can begin to help the child, you might need to call the electric company to turn off the current or the fire department to evaluate toxic fumes.

Look around to gather clues about what might have happened. For instance, there might be a child lying on the ground or below an open second-story window (Figure 2-1 ▶).

Check the scene for more than one injured or ill child. Are all the children in your care present and accounted for? Are there any injured or ill children that have gone unnoticed?

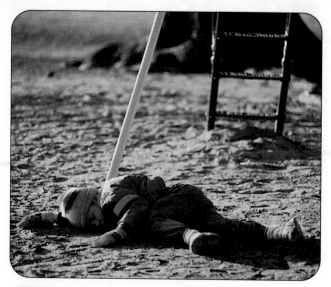

Figure 2-1 Look around to gather clues.

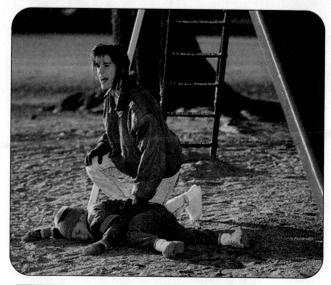

Figure 2-2 Shout for help and send someone to call for emergency medical help.

Calling for Emergency Medical Help

To activate the emergency medical service (EMS) in most communities, simply phone 9-1-1. Check to see if this is true in your community. Emergency telephone numbers are usually listed on the inside cover of telephone directories. Keep your emergency number near or on every telephone. Call the operator using the zero key (0) if you do not know the emergency number.

When you call for help, a dispatcher will often ask several questions. Speak slowly and clearly when you provide this information:

- Your name and the phone number where you are
- Location of the injured or ill child
- What happened
- Number of children needing help
- Child's condition (eg, "Bleeding heavily from the head") and any care that is being provided.

Do not hang up the phone until the dispatcher instructs you to do so. Some EMS systems have an enhanced 9-1-1 phone system that can automatically track a call to its location. But because the location of a cell phone cannot be tracked automaticaly, it is important to convey all of the information and provide a call back number. Also, the dispatcher may be able to tell you how best to care for the child. If you send someone else to make the call have the person report back to you so you know that the call was made.

Initial Assessment: Checking for Life-Threatening Conditions

Perform an initial assessment to find any life-threatening conditions that require immediate attention (**Skill Scan ▶**). Most injuries do not involve life-threatening situations. In most instances, it will take only moments to complete the initial assessment. To perform an initial assessment:

Check responsiveness. If the child does not respond when called by name or gently tapped on the shoulder, assume that the child is unresponsive (unconscious). Send someone to call EMS if the child is unresponsive or appears to have a serious injury or illness (**▲ Figure 2-2**).

Position an unresponsive child on his or her back. Avoid any twisting motion by rolling the head, neck, and spine as a unit.

Check the Airway. Is the airway open? The passageway connecting the nose and mouth to the lungs must be open for air to pass through. If an unresponsive child is positioned flat on the back, the tongue can block the airway. Tilting the head backward slightly moves the tongue out of the airway. Sometimes a foreign object is the cause of a blocked airway.

Check Breathing. Is the child breathing? Breathing supplies oxygen to the heart and other vital organs. When breathing stops, the heart continues to beat for only a few minutes before it, too, stops. To determine if the child is breathing, look, listen, and feel for signs of breathing. If the child is not breathing, you will have to begin rescue breathing. This skill is discussed in detail in Chapter 3.

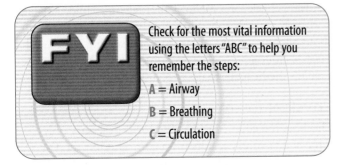

FYI Check for the most vital information using the letters "ABC" to help you remember the steps:

A = Airway

B = Breathing

C = Circulation

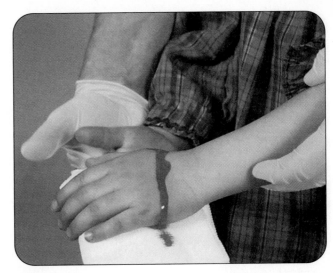

Figure 2-3 A sign is something that can be seen, heard, or felt.

Check Circulation. Once you have checked the child's airway and breathing and corrected any problems, check the child's circulation. Look for signs of normal circulation—breathing, coughing, movement, and normal skin color and temperature. You should also search for and correct any severe bleeding. If the child does not have any signs of circulation, then you must start CPR. This skill is discussed in detail in Chapter 3.

If you suspect a possible spine injury, such as after a fall from a ladder that has caused loss of consciousness or after a motor vehicle accident, try not to move the child. Move the child only as much as is necessary to check the ABCs and perform the care necessary, because any change of position might make the spine injury worse. See Chapter 7: Head and Spine Injuries for the best way to care for a suspected spinal injury.

Checking for Other Problems

Check for other problems only after you are certain that the child does not have any immediate life-threatening problems (ABCs). Now you can locate and prioritize additional problems that do not pose an immediate threat to life but might become life-threatening if left untreated. Often an injury is obvious, such as bleeding or swelling, but you must not assume that the obvious injuries are the only injuries. Most injuries are accompanied by pain and abnormal function.

Help the child to calm down by speaking to the child in a comforting manner. Use short sentences and familiar words. Ask other adults and children if they saw what happened. Reassure the child by explaining that you will help.

Ask simple, nonthreatening questions such as, "Tell me what happened," and, "Point to where it hurts." Try to be as honest as possible. You might not know the extent of the injuries, but you can say, "You are safe now," and "I am taking good care of you." The word SAMPLE can

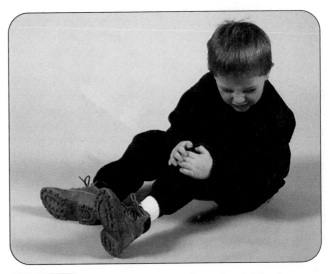

Figure 2-4 A symptom is something the child tells you.

help you remember other important information that EMS may later need.

S: Signs and symptoms are what you observe and the child's complaints (▲ Figures 2-3 and 2-4).

A: Allergies might give a clue to the problem.

M: Medications might give a clue to the problem.

P: Pre-existing condition means a known health condition relating to the problem.

L: Last food or beverage should be known, in case surgery is needed or food poisoning is suspected.

E: Events before the injury, such as a child on playground equipment or eating, can provide clues to the problem.

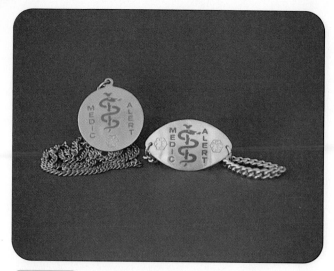

Figure 2-5   Medical alert tag.

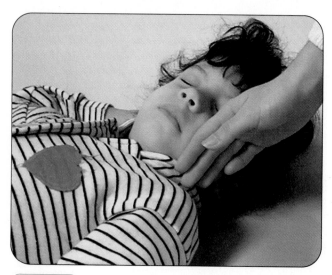

Figure 2-6   Checking body temperature.

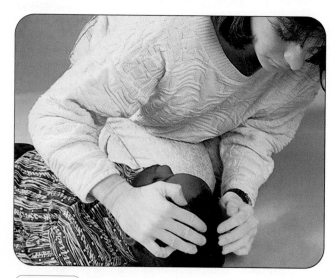

Figure 2-7   Checking the head.

Always check for a medical alert tag on a child. The tag is worn as a necklace or a bracelet. It provides information about allergies, medications, and pre-existing illness and has a 24-hour emergency telephone number. Never remove a child's medical alert tag (◄ Figure 2-5).

Physical Exam

Checking the child from head to toe is necessary only if the child's injury results from a forceful impact. For example, a child might need a head-to-toe check if the child fell from a tree limb or a bicycle or was involved in a motor vehicle crash. In most cases, the child will be able to tell you where the problem is located, and you can direct your attention to that area of the body.

As you examine the child, look for important signs and symptoms of injury. A *sign* is a condition that you see, hear, or feel, such as bleeding, difficulty breathing, or cool skin. A *symptom* is a condition that the child feels and describes to you, such as nausea or pain.

Explain what you are doing and why. Removing clothing is usually not necessary. Always handle an injured child gently and as little as possible. Avoid any unnecessary movements that might aggravate an undetected injury.

Skin Color

A close check of the skin may reveal blue or gray color around a child's lips and nose that indicates the child is having a problem breathing. This may be easily noticed in a light-skinned child, but not as easily seen in a dark-skinned child. For any skin type, color changes can best be seen by looking at the nailbeds or the mucous membranes inside the mouth and the lower eyelids. Healthy mucous membranes are moist and pink because of their many blood vessels. Mucous membranes that do not have enough oxygen appear pale or blue/gray.

Breathing

Once the child calms down, notice if breathing seems difficult or causes pain or discomfort. Does the child use abdominal muscles to breathe or do the nostrils flare?

Temperature

You can get some idea of the child's temperature by touching the back of your hand to the child's cheek, chest, or abdomen (◄ Figure 2-6).

A child with a fever feels unusually warm in these areas. Do not use your fingertips or palm because they are not sensitive to slight temperature differences. If you suspect that a child has a fever, take the child's temperature using a thermometer.

Head

Check the scalp for a bleeding wound, swelling, or depressions (◄ Figure 2-7).

Skill Scan Initial Assessment

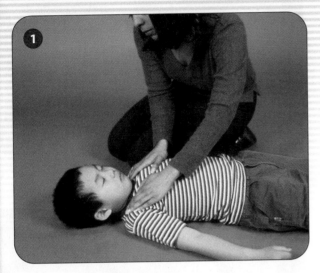

1. Checking responsiveness.

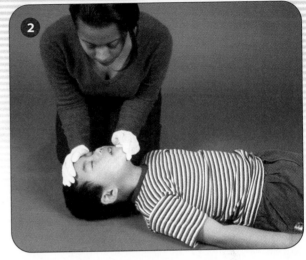

2. A = Airway open? Head tilt–chin lift.

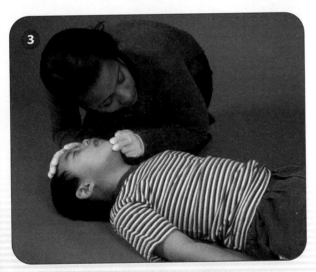

3. B = Breathing? Look, listen, and feel.

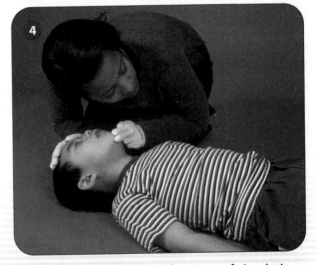

4. C = Circulation? Check for signs of circulation.

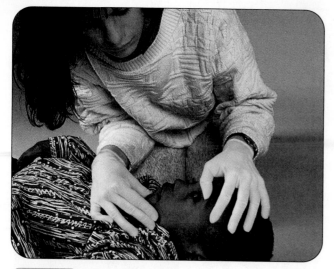

Figure 2-8 Checking the pupils.

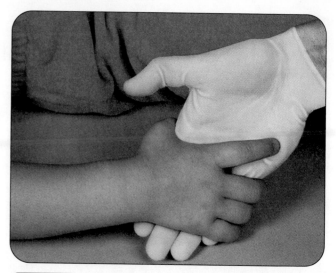

Figure 2-9 Checking for a spinal injury.

Does the child complain of pain? Taking care not to move the head, check the ears and nose for clear fluid or bloody drainage.

Eyes

Gently separate the eyelids and look at the pupils, the small dark centers of the eyes (▲ Figure 2-8).

Normally, pupils become smaller when exposed to light. If the pupils are unequal in size, the child might have experienced an internal head injury. Large or dilated pupils might indicate shock or internal bleeding. Pupils that are constricted might indicate a drug overdose or poisoning.

Spine

Tell the child not to move if you suspect the child has suffered a spine injury. Ask if the child feels any pain or tingling in the arms or legs. Check for sensation (feeling), movement, and strength in the arms and legs by asking the child to wiggle the fingers and toes, to press each foot against your hand, and to squeeze your fingers with each hand (▶ Figures 2-9 and 2-10).

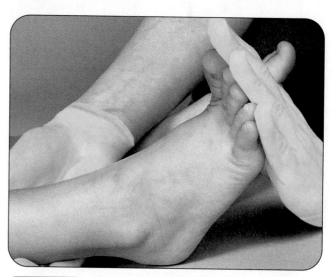

Figure 2-10 Checking for a spinal injury.

Chest

Check for cuts, bruises, penetrations, pain, or unusual positioning of the shoulders and ribs (▶ Figure 2-11).

Abdomen

Gently feel the child's abdomen to check for pain and involuntary tightening of the stomach muscles, called "guarding."

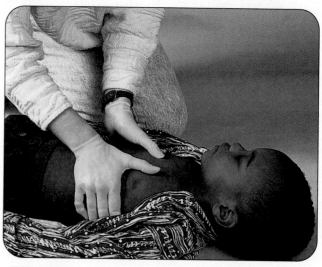

Figure 2-11 Checking the chest and abdomen.

Arms and Legs

Check the child's arms and legs for bleeding, deformity, and pain. Compare one side of the body to the other. The child should be able to move and feel the fingers and toes. The hands and feet should be warm to the touch.

Positioning an Injured or Ill Child

When a serious condition exists, proper positioning makes a child more comfortable, reduces the risk of further injury, and helps prevent the child's condition from worsening. Position the child according to the problems you find and the child's complaints.

Recovery Position

Use this position for a child who is unresponsive but breathing, and for any child who is vomiting. Roll the child onto his or her side as one unit. This position stabilizes and prevents the child from rolling forward or backward. It keeps the airway open and reduces the risk of the child choking on vomit (▶ Figure 2-12).

Raised Head and Shoulders Position

Use this position if the child is experiencing difficulty breathing, but do not use this position if you suspect a spine injury. Elevate the head and shoulders so that the child is in a semi-sitting position, which makes breathing easier (▶ Figure 2-13).

Shock Position

Use this position if the child is exhibiting signs and symptoms of shock or if the seriousness of the problem causes you to think the child might go into shock. Lay the child flat on the back, using blankets or jackets to raise the feet 8" to 12", but no more. This helps to increase the flow of blood to the heart and brain. Use this position only if you do not suspect a spine injury (▶ Figure 2-14).

See Chapter 5 for detailed information on shock.

Moving Children

A seriously ill or injured child should not be moved until he or she is ready for transport to a hospital, if required.

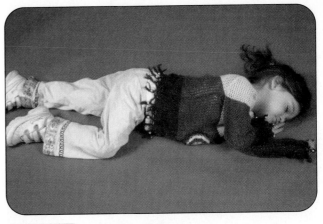

Figure 2-12   Recovery position.

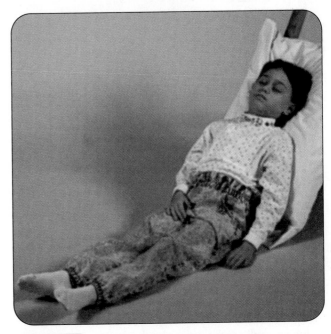

Figure 2-13   Raised head and shoulders position.

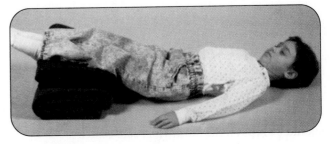

Figure 2-14   Shock position.

If the child is in immediate danger, such as lying near flames, an environment of toxic fumes, or other dangerous environment, the child should be moved to safety in a way that minimizes the risk of further injury.

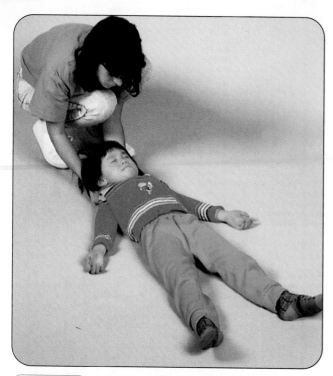

Figure 2-15) Shoulder drag.

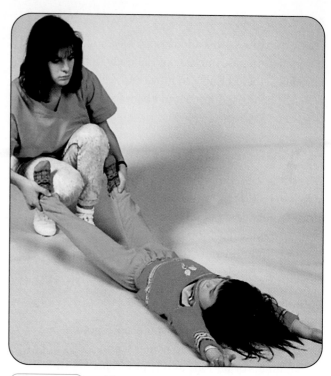

Figure 2-16) Ankle drag.

The major danger in moving a child quickly is the possibility of aggravating an existing problem. If you must do an emergency move, and you suspect a possible spine injury, pull the child in the direction of the long axis of the body to minimize further injury to the spine ▲ Figure 2-15). If a child is on the ground, you can drag the child away from the scene by using various techniques ▲ Figure 2-16).

Methods of moving a child without a spinal injury include a cradle carry and a piggyback carry ▶ Figure 2-17).

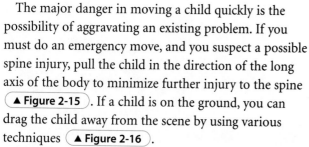

Documentation

If an injury or illness occurs to a child in your child care setting, it is important to document the nature of the injury and the care provided. This information should be kept on file in the child care center.

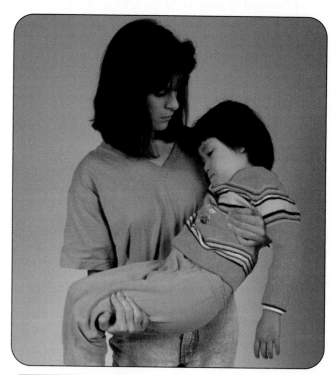

Figure 2-17) Cradle carry.

Documenting an Illness

Date and time illness noted: _____

Child's activity at time of illness: _____

Signs and symptoms of illness: _____

Skin:

_____ Pale   _____ Flushed   _____ Cold, moist   _____ Dry, hot

_____ Blue lips   _____ Blue nail beds   _____ Rash present

Describe rash: _____

Breathing:

_____ Normal   _____ Painful breathing _____ Using abdominal muscles

_____ Wheezing   _____ Tight chest   _____ Coughing   _____ Nasal flaring

Temperature:

Temperature reading: _____ How temperature was taken (oral, rectal, under arm, ear, forehead tape): _____

Child's complaint: _____

Description of care given: _____

Care given by: _____

Was EMS notified? _____ Was the child's health care provider notified? _____

Staff person supervising the child at the time of the illness: _____

Child's parent notified: _____

Date: _____ Time: _____

Signature of person preparing this form: _____

Documenting an Injury

Child's name: _____ Birth date: _____

Date and time of injury: _____

Place where injury occurred: _____

Description of injury: _____

Description of how injury occurred: _____

Description of first aid care given: _____

First aid care given by: _____

Was EMS notified? _____ Was the child's health care provider notified? _____

Adult witness to the injury: _____

Staff person supervising the child at the time of the injury: _____

Child's parent notified: _____

Date: _____ Time: _____

Signature of person preparing this form: _____

Learning Activities

Finding Out What's Wrong

Directions: Circle Yes if you agree with the statement, and circle No if you disagree.

Yes No **1.** A child's medical alert tag should never be removed.

Yes No **2.** A sign is a condition that the child feels.

Yes No **3.** Always begin first aid care with a head-to-toe check.

Yes No **4.** Before approaching an injury scene, make sure that it is safe for you to approach.

Yes No **5.** Healthy mucous membranes are moist and pink.

Yes No **6.** The recovery position is used for a child who is unresponsive and not breathing.

Yes No **7.** A broken bone is usually not a life-threatening emergency.

Yes No **8.** A child with difficulty breathing should be placed in the shock position.

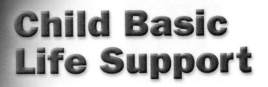

Chapter 3

Child Basic Life Support

Child Rescue Breathing and CPR

Basic Life Support includes rescue breathing, CPR, and care for airway obstruction. Providing basic life support is the most important contribution you can make to another person's welfare. Normal breathing and a beating heart are essential for sustaining life. They are so intimately connected that if one stops, the other also stops.

Cardiopulmonary resuscitation, or CPR, is the care provided when the vital functions of breathing and heartbeat stop. Cardio refers to the heart and pulmonary refers to the lungs.

When the heart stops, all body functions, including breathing, also stop. CPR is a technique that combines chest compressions on the breastbone, or sternum, with breathing into another person's lungs to reproduce the work of the heart and lungs. CPR keeps oxygenated blood circulating to the vital organs—the heart, lungs, and brain.

Another technique, known as rescue breathing, is necessary when only the breathing stops. When breathing stops, the heart continues to beat for a few minutes. But without a continuous supply of oxygen, the heart will stop too. If rescue breathing is started immediately after breathing stops, there is a good chance of preventing the heart from stopping. A bystander can perform either rescue breathing or CPR to keep oxygenated blood circulating to the vital organs until EMS arrives.

Who Needs CPR?

The health problems that first come to mind when thinking about the need for CPR are heart attacks and strokes. Middle-aged and elderly adults who experience sudden death from some form of heart or artery disease are clearly the largest group who benefit from CPR techniques.

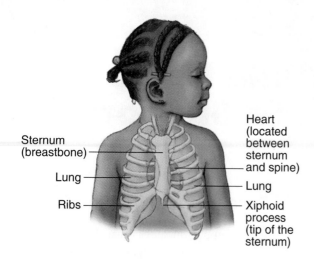

Sternum (breastbone)

Lung

Ribs

Heart (located between sternum and spine)

Lung

Xiphoid process (tip of the sternum)

Figure 3-1 Location of heart and lungs.

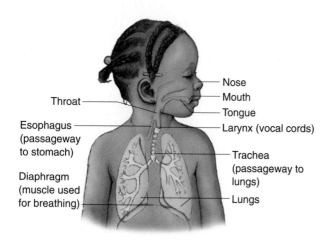

Throat

Esophagus (passageway to stomach)

Diaphragm (muscle used for breathing)

Nose

Mouth

Tongue

Larynx (vocal cords)

Trachea (passageway to lungs)

Lungs

Figure 3-2 The respiratory system.

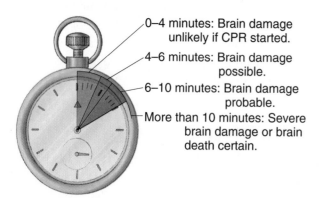

0–4 minutes: Brain damage unlikely if CPR started.

4–6 minutes: Brain damage possible.

6–10 minutes: Brain damage probable.

More than 10 minutes: Severe brain damage or brain death certain.

Figure 3-3

But what about children? For most children, the heart is a healthy, strong muscle pumping blood through unobstructed blood vessels. When a healthy child's heart stops beating, it is seldom caused by a problem within the heart. Instead, the reason is likely an injury that causes the breathing to stop first. Some injuries that could cause a child's breathing to stop are: electrocution, near-drowning, poisoning, smoke inhalation, severe trauma or head injury, and choking.

The Heart, Lung, and Brain Connection

All body tissues need oxygen to live. Oxygen enters the body through the lungs, where it passes into the blood. The heart then circulates this oxygen-rich blood to every cell in the body. Your heart is a muscle about the size of your fist located in the center of your chest behind the sternum. The lungs lie on either side of the heart. Both heart and lungs are protected by the rib cage ◄ **Figures 3-1 and 3-2** .

The most demanding user of oxygen is the brain, the master control center of the body. The brain can survive without oxygen for only 4 to 6 minutes before the risk of brain damage becomes probable. The heart, too, can be damaged if it does not receive oxygen. This is why respiratory arrest (when breathing stops) and cardiac arrest (when the heart stops) are the most urgent life-threatening emergencies ◄ **Figure 3-3** .

CPR can circulate enough oxygen to keep the brain and heart functioning. The air we inhale contains 21% oxygen. The body uses the oxygen it needs and then exhales air that contains 16% oxygen. If this air is breathed into another person's lungs, it still has sufficient oxygen to keep that person's heart, lungs, and brain functioning.

The regular beating of the healthy heart pumps blood throughout the body with high efficiency. When the heart stops beating, external compression of the heart through CPR can restore 25% to 30% of the normal blood circulation. Even though CPR is not as efficient as normal breathing and circulation, it can be sufficient to sustain vital organs in an emergency. In the event of cardiac and respiratory arrest, promptness in starting CPR can determine the quality of life that will be enjoyed by the ill or injured person after recovery.

Barrier Devices for Rescue Breathing

Infant-size or child-size barrier devices for rescue breathing have a one-way valve ▶ Figures 3-4 and 3-5 . These barrier devices should be included in your first aid kit for use in a respiratory or cardiac emergency.

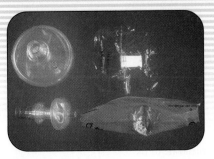

Figure 3-4

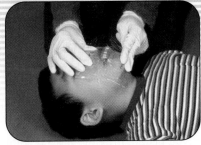

Figure 3-5

Keeping a Heart Healthy

The number 1 killer of Americans is heart disease. Although heart disease is usually seen in adults, routine blood cholesterol screening of grade school children shows that high blood cholesterol levels are already present for some children. These high cholesterol levels are known to contribute to heart disease. For many people, lifestyle changes, such as diet and exercise, can reduce these levels and reduce the chance of developing heart disease later in life.

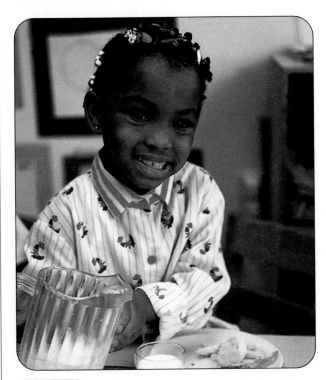

Figure 3-6   Healthy food builds healthy bodies.

Both parents and child care providers are in a position to influence the behaviors, attitudes, and habits of young children in a positive way. Be a good role model and teach these heart-healthy habits:

Teach children not to smoke. If you smoke, avoid doing so in front of children or in an area where children and other staff will breathe the smoke. Both smokers and nonsmokers should be aware of the dangers of smoking. Teach children that it is unhealthy to smoke cigarettes. Consider stopping smoking for yourself and for the people who love you.

Teach children to eat healthy foods. A lifetime of poor dietary habits, especially high-fat diets, can contribute to heart disease. Children need to eat a variety of foods including cereals, breads, pasta, vegetables, fruits, low-fat dairy products, poultry, fish, and lean meats ◀ Figure 3-6 . Fats and sweets, although enjoyable, should be eaten sparingly. Talk about healthy foods at mealtimes and compliment the good choices that children make. If you eat with the children, be sure your meal is heart-healthy.

Teach children to exercise. Most young children enjoy physical activity. Those who remain physically active over the years will reap the benefits as adults. Teach children that activities like running, swimming, outdoor games, riding bicycles, and jumping rope keep their heart muscles strong and healthy.

School-age children and adolescents also need to learn about controlling the additional factors of blood pressure and weight.

Open the Airway

The most common cause of airway obstruction in an unresponsive child is blockage by the tongue. When the child's airway is opened, the lower jaw moves forward, bringing the base of the tongue forward and away from the back of the throat. The easiest way to open the airway is by tilting the head back and lifting the chin. This is done by placing one hand on the child's forehead and two fingers of the other hand under the lower edge of the chin.

If you believe the child has a possible spinal injury, use the jaw thrust technique without head tilt to open the airway. Stabilize the child's head, place your fingers behind the angles of the child's lower jaw on each side of the head, and move the lower jaw forward without tilting the head backward.

Breathing

With the airway open, check for breathing for up to 10 seconds. Place your ear next to the child's mouth, and your eyes on the child's chest. Look, listen, and feel for any signs of breathing.

Positioning

For an unresponsive breathing child, place him or her in the recovery position (Figure 3-7 ▶). For the non-breathing child, rescue breathing must be started immediately.

Rescue Breathing
Mouth-to-Mouth Method

The mouth-to-mouth method of rescue breathing is a simple, quick, and effective method for an emergency situation. With the airway open, pinch the nose shut, take a breath, and breathe into the child with slow breaths. Each breath should be just enough to make the chest rise.

Mouth-to-Nose Method

Although mouth-to-mouth breathing is successful in the majority of cases, certain complications may necessitate mouth-to-nose rescue breathing. For example, if you cannot open the child's mouth, the teeth are clenched together, you cannot make a good seal around the child's mouth, or the child's mouth is severely injured, then you must use the mouth-to-nose method.

The mouth-to-nose technique is performed like mouth-to-mouth breathing, except that you force your exhaled breath through the child's nose while holding his or her mouth closed with one hand pushing up on the chin.

Mouth-to-Barrier Device

A mouth-to-barrier device is an apparatus that is placed over a child's face as a safety precaution for the rescuer during rescue breathing. There are 2 types of mouth-to-barrier devices:

- Masks. Resuscitation masks are clear, plastic devices that cover the child's mouth and nose. They have a one-way valve so exhaled air from the child does not enter the rescuer's mouth (Figure 3-8 ▶).

- Face shields. These clear plastic devices have a mouthpiece through which the rescuer breathes (Figure 3-9 ▶). Some models have a short airway that is inserted into the child's mouth over the tongue. They are smaller and less expensive than masks, but air can leak around the shield. Also, they cover only the child's mouth, so the nose must be pinched.

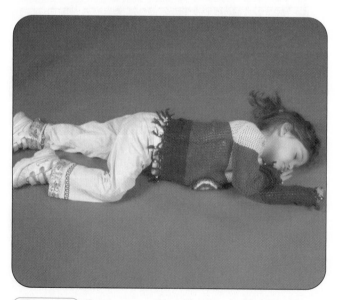

(Figure 3-7) Recovery position. The hand supports the head. Bent knee and arm give stability.

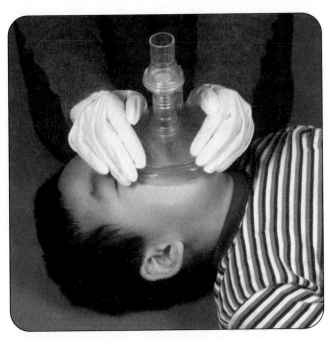

Figure 3-8 Mouth-to-barrier device—mask.

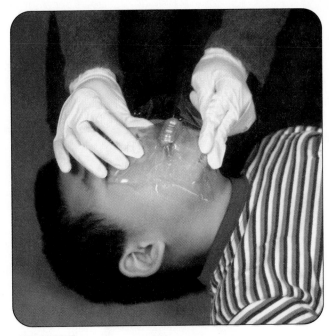

Figure 3-9 Face shield.

After the barrier device is in place, the rescuer breathes through the device. The technique is performed like mouth-to-mouth breathing. See the skill sheets beginning on page 24 for the steps for performing rescue breathing.

Airway Obstruction (Choking)
Recognizing Choking

A foreign body lodged in the airway may cause partial or complete airway obstruction. When a foreign body partially blocks the airway, either good or poor air exchange may result. When good air exchange is present, the child is able to make forceful coughing efforts in an attempt to relieve the obstruction. The child should be permitted and encouraged to cough. Sometimes, however, a good air exchange may progress to a poor air exchange.

A choking child who has poor air exchange has a weak and ineffective cough, and breathing becomes more difficult. The skin, the fingernail beds, and the inside of the mouth may appear bluish-gray in color. Each attempt to inhale is usually accompanied by a high-pitched noise. A partial airway obstruction with poor air exchange should be treated as if it were a complete airway obstruction.

Complete airway obstruction in a responsive child commonly occurs when the child has been eating. Children and infants choke on all kinds of objects. Foods such as

hot dogs, candy, peanuts, and grapes are major offenders because of their shape and consistencies. Non-food choking deaths are caused by balloons, balls, marbles, toys, and coins. With complete airway obstruction, the child is unable to speak, breathe, or cough. When asked, "Can you speak?" the child is unable to respond verbally. Choking children may instinctively reach up and clutch their necks to communicate that they are choking. This motion is known as the distress signal for choking (▼ **Figure 3-10**).

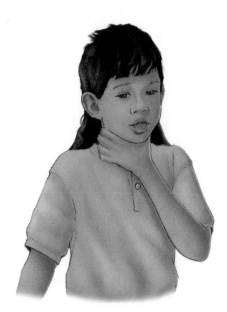

Figure 3-10 Universal sign of choking distress.

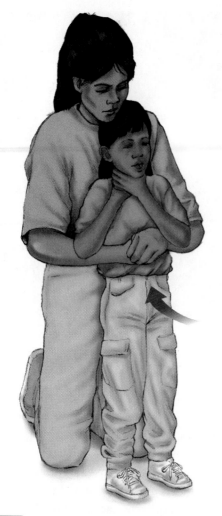

Figure 3-11 Abdominal thrust for a responsive child.

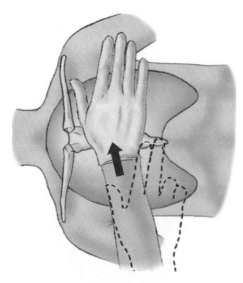

Figure 3-12 Proper hand placement for chest compressions.

The child becomes panicked and desperate and may appear pale in color. Because a complete obstruction prevents air from entering the lungs, brain damage can occur within a few minutes.

Complete airway obstruction in an unresponsive child is usually the result of the tongue relaxing in the back of the mouth, restricting air movement. Proper positioning of the airway can correct this problem.

Care for Choking

Giving abdominal thrusts to a choking child can dislodge the foreign body from the airway. To give abdominal thrusts, position yourself behind the child. Place your arms around the child's waist and form a fist with one hand. Place the thumb side of the fist against the child's abdomen slightly above the navel. With your other hand, hold your fist, and give quick upward and inward thrusts to the child's abdomen (◄ Figure 3-11). See the skill sheet on page 26 for the steps for clearing an airway obstruction.

Cardiopulmonary Resuscitation (CPR)

When the heart stops pumping blood, the child immediately loses consciousness and is considered clinically dead. When this occurs, the heart is not pumping blood and there are only about four minutes to correct this problem before irreversible brain damage occurs. Without intervention, the child will become biologically (irreversibly) dead within minutes. When a child's heart stops beating, he or she needs CPR to be started promptly. CPR is the process of giving rescue breaths and chest compressions to move oxygen throughout the child's body.

Chest compressions are performed with one hand (child 1-8 years). The desired position on the chest is between the nipples, on the lower half of the sternum (◄ Figure 3-12).

For chest compressions to be effective, the child must be on a firm, flat surface. See the skill sheets beginning on page 24 for detailed CPR procedures.

Types of Upper Airway Obstruction

+ **Tongue.** Unconsciousness produces relaxation of soft tissues, and the tongue can fall into the airway. "Swallowing one's tongue" is impossible, but the widespread belief that it can happen is explained by slippage of the relaxed tongue into the airway. The tongue is the most common cause of airway obstruction.

+ **Foreign body.** The National Safety Council reports that more than 2,000 deaths occur in the United States each year because of foreign body airway obstruction. People, especially children, inhale all kinds of objects. Foods such as hotdogs, candy, peanuts, and grapes are major offenders because of their shapes and consistencies. Balloons are the top cause of nonfood choking deaths in children, followed by balls, marbles, toys, and coins. Unconscious children's airways also can be obstructed by a foreign body (eg, vomit).

+ **Swelling.** Severe allergic reactions (anaphylaxis) and irritants (eg, smoke, chemicals) can cause swelling. Even a nonallergic person who is stung inside the throat by a bee, yellow jacket, or flying insect can experience swelling in the airway.

+ **Spasm.** Water that is suddenly inhaled can cause a spasm in the throat. This happens in about 10 percent of all drownings. When such a spasm does not allow the lungs to fill with water, it is known as a "dry drowning."

+ **Vomit.** Expect vomiting to occur during CPR.

Basic Life Support
Child Rescue Breathing and CPR

If you see a motionless child …

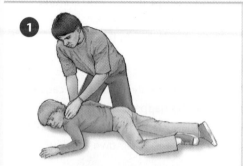

Check responsiveness
- Tap the child and shout, "Are you okay?"
- If unresponsive, go to step #2.

Have someone call the local emergency number, usually 9-1-1.

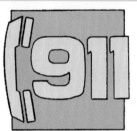

Open airway
- Tilt the head back and lift the chin.
- If you suspect a spinal injury, use jaw-thrust method without head-tilt.

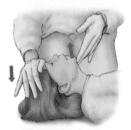
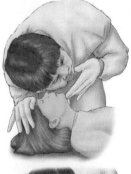
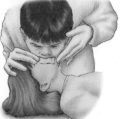

Check breathing (10 seconds)
- Look, listen, and feel for breathing.
- If breathing, place child in recovery position.
- If not breathing, give 2 slow rescue breaths (1–1½ seconds each).
- If breaths do not cause the chest to rise, the airway may be blocked. Reposition the head and try breaths again. If chest does not rise, begin CPR (see step #6). When you open the airway to give a breath, look for an object in the throat and if seen, remove it.
- If breaths cause the chest to rise, continue to step #5.

Basic Life Support
Child Rescue Breathing and CPR

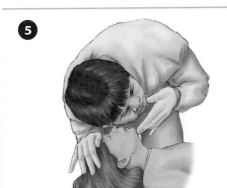

⑤

Check for signs of circulation (10 seconds)
Signs of circulation include:

- Breathing
- Coughing
- Movement
- Normal skin condition
- Responsiveness
- Pulse

If not breathing, but other signs of circulation exist, give 1 breath about every 3 seconds. Recheck signs of circulation every minute.

If no signs of circulation, begin CPR (step #6).

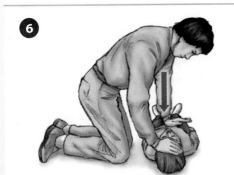

⑥

Perform CPR

- Place heel of 1 hand on the center of the chest between the nipples (lower half of the sternum).
- Place other hand on child's forehead.
- Using 1 hand, depress chest downward 1 to 1½ inches.
- Give 5 chest compressions at a rate of about 100 per minute.
- Open the airway and give 1 slow breath (1 to 1½ seconds).
- Repeat cycles of 5 chest compressions and 1 rescue breath.

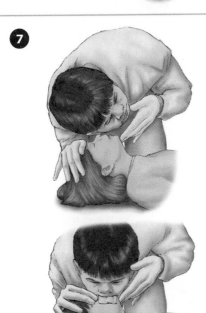

⑦

Recheck circulation

After about 1 minute, recheck for signs of circulation.

- If not breathing and no other signs of circulation exist, resume CPR.
- If breathing, place child in recovery position.
- If not breathing, but other signs of circulation exist, provide 1 rescue breath about every 3 seconds.
- Recheck for signs of circulation every few minutes.

Basic Life Support
Child Airway Obstruction

If child is responsive and cannot speak, breathe or cough...

1

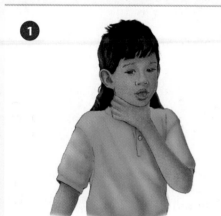

Check child for choking

- Ask, "Are you choking? Can you speak?".
- A choking child cannot speak, breathe, or cough and may clutch the neck with one or both hands.

2

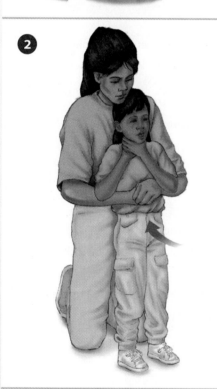

Give abdominal thrusts (Heimlich maneuver)

- Place a fist against the child's abdomen just above the navel.
- Grasp the fist with your other hand and press into child's abdomen with quick inward and upward thrusts.
- Continue thrusts until object is removed or child becomes unresponsive.

3

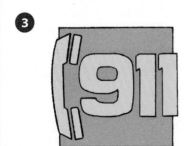

If the child becomes unresponsive

- Have someone call 9-1-1 or emergency telephone number to activate the EMS system.
- Assess the child and begin CPR if needed.
- Each time you open the airway to give a breath, look for an object in the throat and if seen, remove it.

Child Basic Life Support
Proficiency Checklist

S = self check / P = partner check / I = instructor check

Child Rescue Breathing

	S	P	I
1. Check responsiveness.	○	○	○
2. Send a bystander, if available, to call EMS.	○	○	○
3. **A**irway open.	○	○	○
4. **B**reathing check.	○	○	○
5. 2 slow breaths.	○	○	○
6. **C**heck circulation.	○	○	○
7. Rescue breathing (1 every 3 seconds).	○	○	○
8. If alone, call EMS after 1 minute.	○	○	○
9. Recheck circulation and breathing after first minute, then every few minutes.	○	○	○

Child CPR

	S	P	I
1. Check responsiveness.	○	○	○
2. Send a bystander, if available, to call EMS.	○	○	○
3. Airway open.	○	○	○
4. Breathing check.	○	○	○
5. 2 slow breaths.	○	○	○
6. Check circulation.	○	○	○
7. Position hand.	○	○	○
8. 5 compressions with 1 hand.	○	○	○
9. 1 slow breath.	○	○	○
10. Continue CPR for 1 minute (19 more cycles, for total of 20).	○	○	○
11. If alone, call EMS after 1 minute.	○	○	○
12. Recheck circulation.	○	○	○
13. Continue CPR.	○	○	○
14. Recheck circulation every few minutes.	○	○	○

Child Choking

	S	P	I
1. Position hands.	○	○	○
2. Give abdominal thrusts until the object is removed or the child is unresponsive.	○	○	○
3. If unresponsive, assess child and begin CPR if needed.	○	○	○

Learning Activities

Child Basic Life Support

Directions: Circle Yes if you agree with the statement, and circle No if you disagree.

Yes   No   **1.** Child CPR requires 5 compressions and 1 breath.

Yes   No   **2.** An unresponsive, breathing child should be placed in the recovery position.

Yes   No   **3.** When performing rescue breathing, breathe forcefully to make sure the chest rises quickly.

Yes   No   **4.** If a child can cough forcefully, he or she is choking and needs the Heimlich maneuver.

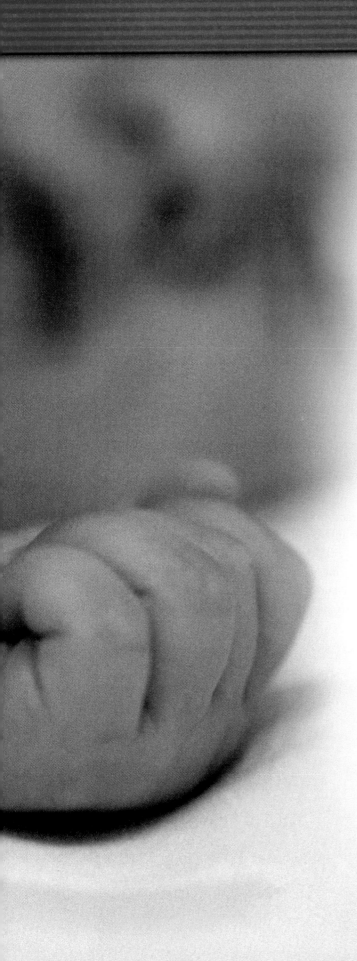

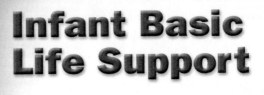

Chapter 4

Infant Basic Life Support

Infant Rescue Breathing and CPR

Basic life support techniques for an infant (under one year) differ only slightly from those for a child (1-8 years) or adult (>8 years). Cardiac arrest in infants, like children, is rare. Cardiac arrest is often secondary to respiratory arrest, because the heart muscle did not receive sufficient oxygen.

Responsiveness

The first priority in cardiopulmonary emergency is to determine the infant's responsiveness. This is done by tapping the infant and speaking loudly. If basic life support is necessary, give resuscitation for one minute before activating the EMS. The rescuer should shout for help to get someone's attention.

Properly position the infant so that if any resuscitation efforts are needed, they can be performed. If the infant is found lying facedown, turn the infant as a complete unit onto his or her back.

A: Airway

After unresponsiveness has been determined and the infant has been properly positioned, open the airway by using the head tilt–chin lift method. To do this, place one hand and apply pressure gently to the infant's forehead to tilt the head backward. Do not overtilt the head backward because it can block the airway because of the pliability of the infant's airway. To lift the chin, place the finger(s) of your other hand under the bony part of the jaw. Then lift your fingers to bring the chin up. The fingers should not press on the soft tissue under the infant's chin because it can interfere with the opening of the airway. While the chin is lifted, the hand on the forehead maintains the head tilt position of the infant. Sometimes, opening the airway may be all that is necessary for the infant to breathe.

When a spinal injury is suspected, open the airway using the jaw thrust without tilting the head back. If the airway remains blocked, tilt the head slowly and gently until the airway is open. This technique for a suspected spinal-injured infant will help minimize any existing injury. While stabilizing the head, place the fingers of each hand behind the angles of the infant's lower jaw on each side of the head and move the lower jaw forward without tilting the head backward; however, it may be necessary to tilt the head slightly if the airway cannot be opened.

B: Breathing

After unresponsiveness has been determined and the airway has been opened, you should look, listen, and feel for breathing. You should (1) look to see whether there is any movement of the infant's chest, (2) listen for air by placing your ear next to the infant's mouth and nose, and (3) feel for air by placing your cheek next to the infant's mouth and nose. If breathing is present, you will see the infant's chest rise and fall, hear air coming from the infant's mouth and nose, and feel air against your cheek.

Rescue Breathing

The breaths for an infant should be limited to the amount needed to raise the chest. For infants, use shallow puffs of air.

To perform rescue breathing for an infant, follow these steps:

1. Open the airway.

2. Form an airtight seal over the infant's nose and mouth (or nose only).

3. Give 2 breaths using shallow puffs of air.

4. Watch to see if the infant's chest rises.

> ### Children and Gastric Distention
>
> Rescue breathing can cause stomach or gastric distention more often in infants and children than in adults. Minimize this problem by limiting the breaths to the amount needed to make the chest rise. Avoid overinflating the lungs. Gastric distention can cause regurgitation and aspiration of stomach contents.

5. Between breaths, remove your mouth from the infant's to allow air to flow out of the infant's lungs.

If breaths do not go in, reposition the head. If they still do not go in, begin CPR as indicated in the skill sheets beginning on page 33.

If the infant is not breathing, but has other signs of circulation, continue rescue breathing. Because infants breathe faster than adults, breathe into an infant once every 3 seconds or 20 times a minute. Between breaths, remove your mouth from the infant's to allow air to flow out of the infant's lungs. As you remove your mouth, you should turn your head to the side to see if the infant's chest fell after each breath. For rescue breathing, breathe into the infant with just enough air to make the chest gently rise.

C: Circulation

After an infant has been given 2 breaths, check for signs of circulation.

If breathing is absent, but other signs of circulation exist, continue rescue breathing. A rescue breath is given every 3 seconds or 20 times a minute. After 20 breaths, you should activate EMS.

If there are no signs of circulation, begin CPR. The proper chest compression point on an infant is the mid-sternum. To locate this area, imagine a line connecting the infant's nipples. Place 3 fingers (index, middle, and ring) with the index finger next to but below the imaginary nipple line. Lift the index finger off the chest ▼ Figure 4-1 .

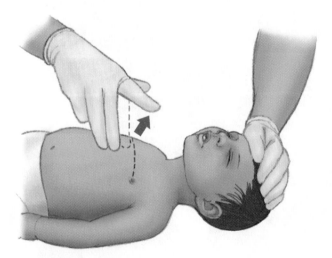

Figure 4-1 Proper finger placement for chest compressions.

Use the 2 remaining fingers to apply the chest compressions. Press the infant's midsternum (area between the nipples) 1/2 to 1 inch into the chest with the middle and ring finger. Either place your other hand under the infant's shoulder to provide support or keep it on the infant's forehead to keep the head tilted. If the infant is carried during CPR, the length of the body is on the rescuer's forearm with the head kept level with the trunk.

An infant's heart rate is faster than an adult's and so the rate of compressions must also be faster. The infant compression rate is at least 100 per minute. External chest compressions must always be combined with rescue breathing. The ratio of compressions to breaths is 5 to 1. See the skill sheets for Infant CPR beginning on page 33 (Skill Scan ▶).

Airway Obstruction (Choking)

As discussed before, the airway may be partially or completely blocked. With a partial airway obstruction, an infant is able to make persistent coughing efforts that should not be hampered. If good air exchange becomes a poor exchange or poor air exchange occurs initially, the infant should be managed as having a complete airway obstruction. Poor air exchanges are indicated by ineffective coughing, high-pitched noises, breathing difficulty, and blueness of the lips and fingernail beds.

Choking management of a completely obstructed airway consists of the combination of back blows and chest thrusts. Abdominal thrusts are not advisable for infants because of possible injury to the abdominal organs. Any visible object can be removed from the mouth using a finger sweep.

Back Blows and Chest Thrusts

To perform back blows on an infant, straddle the infant facedown over your forearm. The infant's head should be lower than the trunk. Your hand should be around the jaw and neck of the infant, giving support to the infant's head. For more support, rest your forearm under the infant on your thigh. Using the heel of the other hand, give 5 back blows between the infant's shoulder blades (▼ Figure 4-2).

To give chest thrusts, turn the infant onto his or her back. After delivering the 5 back blows, immediately place your free hand on the back of the infant's head and neck while the other hand remains in place. Using both hands and forearms to sandwich the infant—1 supporting the jaw, neck, and chest, and the other the back—turn the infant over. Once turned onto the back, the infant should be resting on your thigh. The infant's head should be lower than the trunk. With the infant positioned, give 5 chest thrusts in rapid succession. The thrusts are given to the sternum (between the nipples), using 2 fingers. The technique used to locate and perform thrusts is the same as that used to perform external chest compressions for CPR (▼ Figure 4-3). See the skill sheet for Infant Airway Obstruction on page 37.

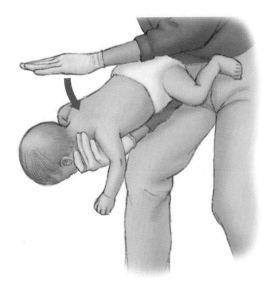
Figure 4-2 Give 5 back blows.

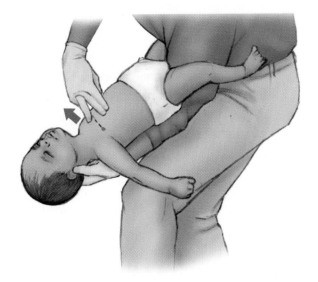
Figure 4-3 Give 5 chest thrusts.

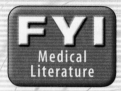

Facts About Sudden Infant Death Syndrome (SIDS)

Many more children die of SIDS in a year than all who die of cancer, heart disease, pneumonia, child abuse, AIDS, cystic fibrosis, and muscular dystrophy combined …

What Is SIDS?

- Sudden Infant Death Syndrome (SIDS) is a medical term that describes the sudden death of an infant that remains unexplained after all known and possible causes have been carefully ruled out through autopsy, death scene investigation, and review of the medical history. SIDS is responsible for more deaths than any other cause in childhood for babies one month to one year of age, claiming 150,000 victims in the United States in this generation alone—7,000 babies each year—*nearly one baby every hour of every day.* It strikes families of all races, ethnic, and socioeconomic origins without warning; neither parent nor physician can predict that something is going wrong. In fact, most SIDS victims appear healthy prior to death.

What Causes SIDS?

- While there are still no adequate medical explanations for SIDS deaths, current theories include: (1) stress in a normal baby, caused by infection or other factors; (2) a birth defect; (3) failure to develop; and/or (4) a critical period when all babies are especially vulnerable, such as a time of rapid growth.

- Many new studies have been launched to learn how and why SIDS occurs. Scientists are exploring the development and function of the nervous system, the brain, the heart, breathing and sleep patterns, body chemical balances, autopsy findings, and environmental factors. It is likely that SIDS, like many other medical disorders, will eventually have more than one explanation.

Can SIDS Be Prevented?

- No, not yet. But, some recent studies have begun to isolate several risk factors that, though not causes of SIDS in and of themselves, may play a role in some cases. (It is important that, since the causes of SIDS remain unknown, SIDS parents refrain from concluding that their child care practices may have caused their baby's death.)

Some Basic Facts about SIDS:

- SIDS is a definite medical entity and is the major cause of death in infants after the first month of life.

- SIDS claims the lives of over 7,000 American babies each year … *nearly one baby every hour of every day.*

- SIDS victims appear to be healthy prior to death.

- Currently, SIDS cannot be predicted or prevented, even by a physician.

- There appears to be no suffering; death occurs very rapidly, usually during sleep.

What SIDS Is Not:

- SIDS is **not** caused by external suffocation.

- SIDS is **not** caused by vomiting and choking.

- SIDS is **not** contagious.

- SIDS does **not** cause pain or suffering in the infant.

- SIDS can**not** be predicted.

Source: SIDS Network. Used with permission.

Basic Life Support
Infant Rescue Breathing and CPR

If you see a motionless infant ...

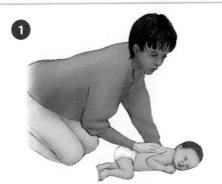

1

Check responsiveness

- Tap the infant and shout, "Are you okay?"

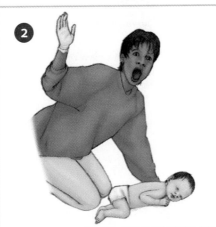

2

Activate EMS

- Have someone call the local emergency telephone number, usually 9-1-1.
- If you are alone, call EMS after 1 minute of resuscitation, unless a bystander can be sent.

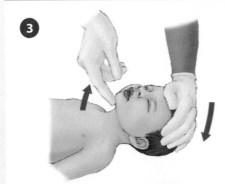

3

Open the airway (use head tilt–chin lift method)

- Place your hand that is nearest infant's head on infant's forehead and tilt head back slightly.
- Place the fingers of your other hand under the chin and lift gently. Avoid pressing on the soft tissues under the jaw.

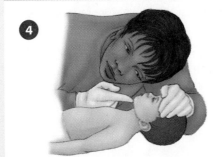

4

Check for breathing (10 seconds)

- Place your ear over the infant's mouth and nose while keeping the airway open.
- *Look* at the infant's chest to check for rise and fall; *listen* and *feel* for breathing.

Basic Life Support
Infant Rescue Breathing and CPR

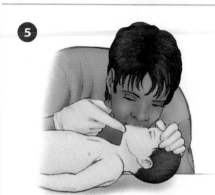

5

If not breathing, give 2 slow breaths

- Keep the airway open.
- Take a breath and place your mouth over the infant's mouth and nose, or nose only.
- Each breath 1–1½ seconds.
- Watch chest rise to see if your breaths go in.
- Allow for chest deflation after each breath.

If breaths do not go in

Retilt the head and try again.

If unsuccessful give CPR. Each time you open the airway, look for an object in the throat, and if seen, remove it.

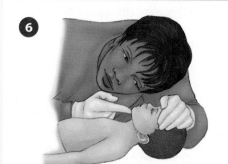

6

Check for signs of circulation (10 seconds)

Signs of circulation include:

- Breathing
- Coughing
- Movement
- Normal skin condition
- Responsiveness
- Pulse

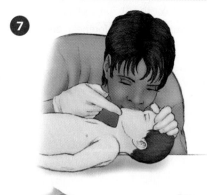

7

If no breathing, but other signs of circulation present

- Give 1 breath every 3 seconds.
- Recheck signs of circulation every minute.

If there are no signs of circulation

- Begin CPR.
    1. Place 2-3 fingers in the center of the chest.
    2. Compress the chest 5 times.
    3. Push sternum straight down ½ to 1 inch.
    4. Compress the chest at a rate of at least 100 compressions per minute.
- Give 1 slow breath.
- Continue cycles of 5 compressions and 1 breath for 1 minute, then check for signs of circulation. If absent, restart CPR with chest compressions. Recheck the signs of circulation every few minutes. If there are signs of circulation but no breathing, give rescue breathing.

Basic Life Support
Infant Airway Obstruction

If infant is responsive and cannot cry, breathe or cough…

1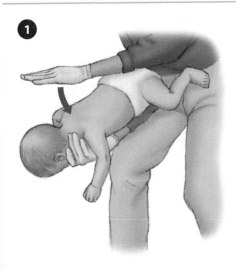

Give up to 5 back blows

- Hold the infant's head and neck with 1 hand by firmly supporting the infant's jaw between your thumb and fingers.

- Lay the infant facedown over your forearm with head lower than his or her chest. Brace your forearm and the infant against your thigh.

- Give up to 5 distinct and separate back blows between the infant's shoulder blades with the heel of your hand.

2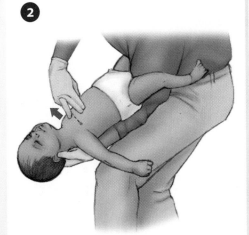

Give up to 5 chest thrusts

- While supporting the back of the infant's head, roll the infant face up.

- Place 3 fingers on the infant's sternum with your ring finger next to and below the imaginary nipple line toward the infant's feet.

- Lift your ring finger off the chest.

- Give up to 5 separate and distinct thrusts with your index and middle fingers on the infant's sternum in a manner similar to CPR chest compressions, but at a slower rate.

3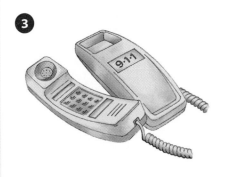

Repeat

- Until the infant becomes unresponsive. Call 9-1-1, assess the infant, and begin CPR if needed. Each time you open the airway to give a breath, look for an object in the throat and if seen, remove it.

OR

- Until the object is expelled, and infant begins to breathe or cough forcefully.

Infant Basic Life Support Proficiency Checklist

S = self check / P = partner check / I = instructor check

Infant Rescue Breathing

	S	P	I
1. Check responsiveness.	○	○	○
2. Send a bystander, if available, to call EMS.	○	○	○
3. Airway open.	○	○	○
4. Breathing check.	○	○	○
5. 2 slow breaths.	○	○	○
6. Check circulation.	○	○	○
7. Rescue breathing (1 every 3 seconds).	○	○	○
8. If alone, call EMS after 1 minute.	○	○	○
9. Recheck circulation and breathing after first minute, then every few minutes.	○	○	○

Infant CPR

	S	P	I
1. Check responsiveness.	○	○	○
2. Send a bystander, if available, to call EMS.	○	○	○
3. Airway open.	○	○	○
4. Breathing check.	○	○	○
5. 2 slow breaths.	○	○	○
6. Check circulation.	○	○	○
7. Position fingers.	○	○	○
8. 5 compressions with 2–3 fingers.	○	○	○
9. 1 slow breath.	○	○	○
10. Continue CPR for 1 minute.	○	○	○
11. If alone, call EMS after 1 minute.	○	○	○
12. Recheck circulation.	○	○	○
13. Continue CPR.	○	○	○
14. Recheck circulation every few minutes.	○	○	○

Infant Choking

	S	P	I
1. 5 back blows.	○	○	○
2. 5 chest thrusts until the object is removed or the infant is unresponsive.	○	○	○
3. If unresponsive, assess infant, give CPR if needed.	○	○	○

Differences Between Adult (>8 years) and Child (1 – 8 years) Basic Life Support

IF adult (>8 years) ...	THEN ...
Is unresponsive and rescuer is alone	activate EMS immediately after determining unresponsiveness.
Is *not* breathing but other signs of circulation exist	• give *2 second breaths.* • give *1 breath every 5 seconds.*
Does *not* have any signs of circulation	• give *chest compressions with 2 hands* on victim's chest. • give *2 breaths after every 15 chest compressions.*

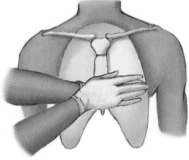

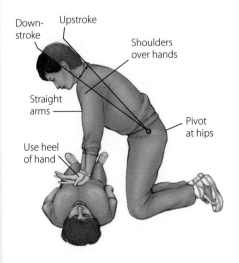

Down-stroke

Upstroke

Shoulders over hands

Straight arms

Pivot at hips

Use heel of hand

Learning Activities

Infant Basic Life Support

Directions: Circle Yes if you agree with the statement, and circle No if you disagree.

Yes   No   **1.** To open an infant's airway, tilt the head back further than you would for an adult.

Yes   No   **2.** Abdominal thrusts are used to clear an airway obstruction in an infant.

Yes   No   **3.** Breathing emergencies are more common than cardiac emergencies in infants.

Yes   No   **4.** During infant CPR, compress the chest $1/2$ to 1 inch, at a rate of at least 100 times per minute.

Yes   No   **5.** If you are alone, provide one minute of care for a nonbreathing infant before calling EMS.

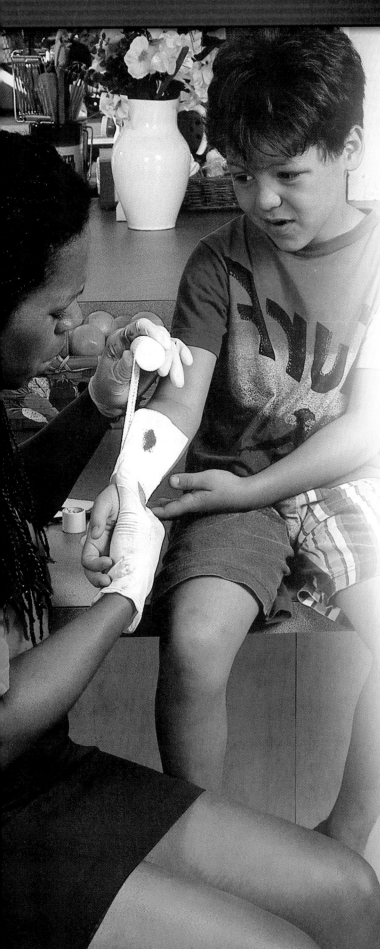

Chapter 5

Bleeding and Shock

Types of Bleeding

When the skin is cut and a blood vessel of any size is broken, bleeding occurs. The seriousness of the injury is determined by how deep the cut is, the type of blood vessels damaged, the amount of bleeding that occurs, and the time it takes to control it.

The most severe bleeding is from arteries, which are large, deep and well-protected blood vessels. Injury to an artery is serious. Arteries carry blood away from the heart to all parts of the body under the strong pressure exerted by each heartbeat. Bright red arterial blood spurts from a damaged artery with each beat of the heart and can be difficult to control—even life-threatening.

Veins are blood vessels that carry blood back to the heart. They are located closer to the surface of the skin than arteries. Bleeding from veins is slower than from arteries because the blood is under less pressure. Although a vein can bleed heavily, it can usually be controlled with simple first aid measures. Venous blood is dark red in color.

Tiny blood vessels located throughout the body are called capillaries. There are hundreds of thousands of capillaries throughout the surface of the skin. When broken, their oozing is the most easily controlled.

Some parts of the body have more blood vessels than others. For example, the head and face have an abundance of blood vessels, so a cut there bleeds profusely.

Open Wounds

When a child has an open wound, the first concern is to stop the bleeding. Once you do that, a fresh wound remains, which, if properly cared for, will heal in a timely fashion. Sometimes a wound can appear to be more serious than it actually is because of the amount of bleeding. Once bleeding is controlled you can see the wound and more accurately determine how serious it is.

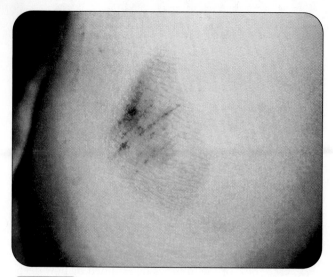

Figure 5-1 Abrasion.

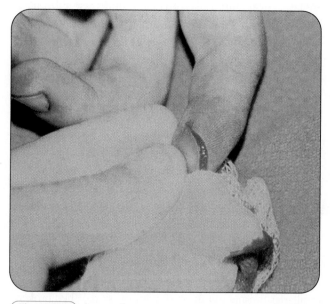

Figure 5-2 Laceration.

Tetanus

Tetanus is a grave disease that causes strong, painful spasms in the back, arms, legs, and jaw—hence its other name, "lockjaw." The disease is usually fatal. Fortunately, however, because of widespread immunization, most residents of the United States are immune to the disease; in this country, there are only about 100 deaths from tetanus each year, far below the world average.

Tetanus bacteria live in soil, dust, and human and animal feces. They are usually introduced into the human body by a sharp object that pierces the skin, but they can enter through any opening in the skin that becomes contaminated with material containing the bacteria. Puncture wounds, because they can be deep and are difficult to clean, are the most likely wounds to become infected with tetanus bacteria. Furthermore, puncture wounds close, and tetanus bacteria are trapped inside where they thrive in an environment with little or no oxygen. In this environment, tetanus bacteria produce a toxin that attacks the central nervous system and brain.

Tetanus can be completely prevented through immunization. Immunization enables the immune system to manufacture its own antitoxin against a future exposure to tetanus. Children should receive a series of five tetanus immunization injections by the age of 6. They should receive a booster in the early adolescent years, and then every 10 years thereafter. Immunizations are the best defense against tetanus.

Common open wounds you may encounter include:

- Abrasion—Top layer of skin is removed, with little blood loss. An example of an abrasion is a scraped knee (▲ **Figure 5-1**).
- Laceration—A cut which could be jagged or smooth. An example of a laceration is a glass or paper cut (▲ **Figure 5-2**).
- Puncture—Often a deep, narrow wound, with a high risk of infection. An example of a puncture wound is a tack or staple in a finger.

Dressings and Bandages

A dressing is a clean covering placed over a wound. A bandage holds the dressing in place and applies pressure to help control bleeding. An adhesive bandage (eg, BAND-AID) is a combination of a dressing and a bandage. For many children, a colorful adhesive bandage can go a long way toward easing the upset caused by a minor skin wound. A larger wound, however, often needs a separate dressing and a bandage.

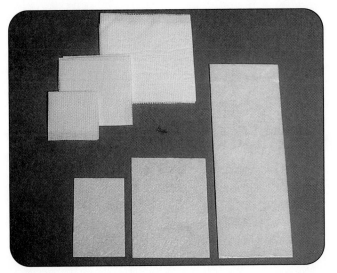

Figure 5-3 Gauze pads used for wound dressings.

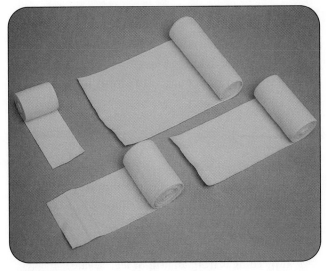

Figure 5-5 Elastic bandages used to apply compression to an extremity.

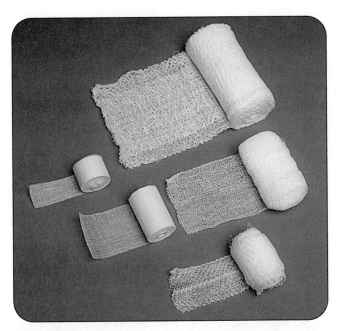

Figure 5-4 Rolled gauze bandages used to hold dressings in place.

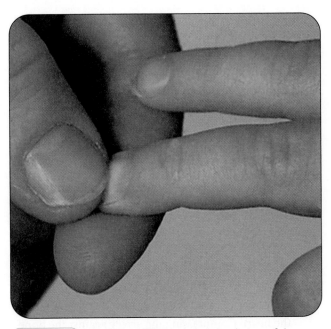

Figure 5-6 Capillary refill: check the circulation of the injured limb by squeezing the nailbed on the limb.

It is best to stock commercial dressings, such as regular gauze pads, nonstick gauze pads, and adhesive bandages, because they come in a variety of sizes, are lint-free, and are packaged sterile (▲ **Figure 5-3**).

A roll of wrapped gauze makes a good bandage because it can be used on any part of the body (▲ **Figure 5-4**).

Elastic bandages provide compression and support to a joint or muscle and can reduce swelling after an injury (▲ **Figure 5-5**). Leave the tips of fingers and toes exposed so that you can tell whether the bandage is wrapped too tightly. Check for changes in color, temperature, and capillary refill in the fingers or toes of the injured limb. They should have normal skin color and feel warm to the touch. Use the capillary refill test to check circulation: firmly squeeze the child's nailbed in the injured limb (▲ **Figure 5-6**). The nailbed should turn white and immediately return to the normal pink color.

External Bleeding

Many children, as well as adults, become anxious at the sight of blood. In most situations, bleeding can be controlled in 5 to 10 minutes with proper first aid.

What to Do

1. Apply firm, direct pressure. Wear disposable gloves and cover the injury with several gauze pads or the cleanest covering available, and press firmly against it for 5 to 10 minutes.

2. If bleeding is from an arm or leg, elevate the injured body part while continuing to apply direct pressure. This uses gravity to slow the flow of blood.

3. Maintain pressure by placing several gauze pads over the bleeding wound and securing them firmly with a roll of gauze or tape, making a pressure bandage. This keeps pressure on the bleeding wound and frees your hands to attend to other injuries. Do not remove the original dressing. If it becomes soaked with blood, add more gauze pads. Removing the original dressing disturbs the blood vessels and interferes with clotting.

4. Apply pressure at a pressure point if severe bleeding cannot be controlled using direct pressure and elevation. A pressure point is located where a main artery passes over a bone between the injury and the heart. Compressing the artery against the bone slows the flow of blood to the bleeding limb. The brachial pressure points control bleeding in the arms and the femoral pressure points do so for the legs.

5. Treat for shock, if necessary.

6. Call for emergency medical help, if necessary. Notify the child's parent.

Barriers Between You and Blood

Coming in contact with blood and other body fluids, such as stool, urine, mucus, and vomit, can allow transmission of organisms such as the hepatitis B virus and HIV. These diseases threaten health and life. Keep a pair of disposable gloves in an easily accessible location, such as your first aid kit. If disposable gloves are not immediately available, use another type of protective barrier to provide a shield between your skin and another person's blood or other body fluids. Barriers also protect a child with an open wound from contaminants on your hands. Examples of protective barriers include:

+ Disposable gloves

+ A plastic bag or anything that is waterproof

+ Several thick layers of gauze pads

+ Clean, thickly folded cloth diaper or dish towel.

About Clotting

Clotting is the process that thickens the blood at the wound site to gradually stop the bleeding and seal the wound. In a small wound, this process takes 3 to 5 minutes to begin after the heavy flow of blood is reduced.

About Stitches

A large deep wound or one that continues to bleed needs to be stitched, or sutured, to reduce the risk of infection, promote healing, and decrease scarring. The size of the wound as well as the location on the body help to determine whether stitches are necessary. This should be decided by a health care provider within 4 to 6 hours after the injury. If more time passes, the edges of the wound begin to heal separately, making it difficult to rejoin them. Without sutures, the wound will heal more slowly, increasing the likelihood of infection and scarring.

Skill Scan   Bleeding Control

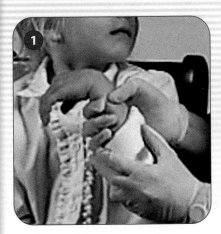

1. Apply direct pressure.

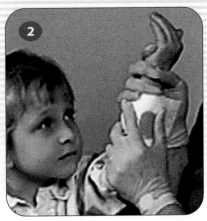

2. Elevate the injured area.

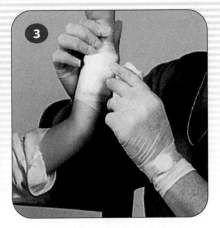

3. Apply a pressure bandage.

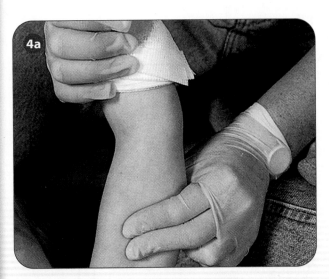

4. Apply pressure to a pressure point:
(a) brachial pressure point,

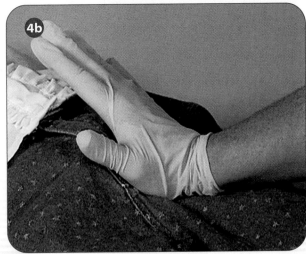

(b) femoral pressure point.

BLEEDING

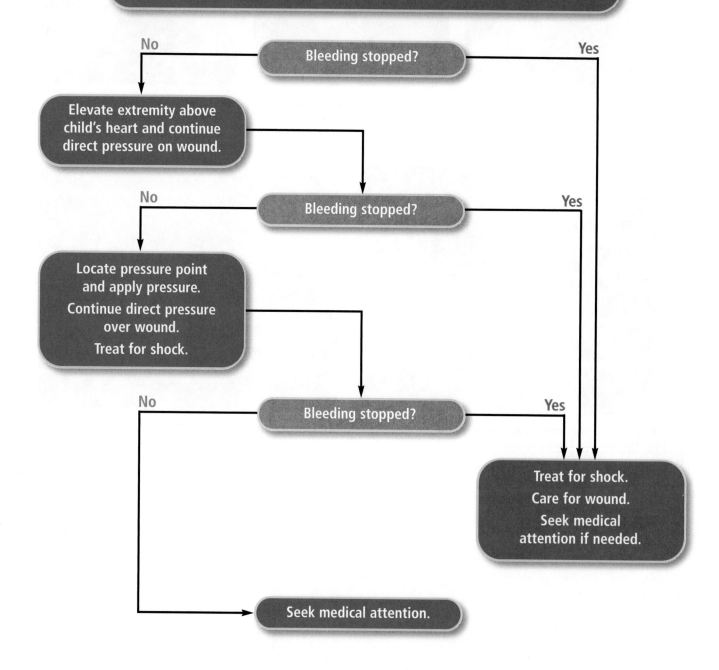

Apply direct pressure over wound
- Place sterile dressing or cleanest cloth available over wound.
- If possible, use medical exam gloves, extra dressing, or plastic wrap.
- *Do not* remove an impaled object.

No — Bleeding stopped? — Yes

Elevate extremity above child's heart and continue direct pressure on wound.

No — Bleeding stopped? — Yes

Locate pressure point and apply pressure.
Continue direct pressure over wound.
Treat for shock.

No — Bleeding stopped? — Yes

Treat for shock.
Care for wound.
Seek medical attention if needed.

Seek medical attention.

Signs of Infection

Occasionally, a healing wound develops an infection that requires medical treatment (▼ **Figure 5-7**). Signs of infection include:

- Throbbing pain

- Swelling

- Pus or other discharge

- Skin red and warm to the touch

- Red streaks leading away from the wound

- Fever

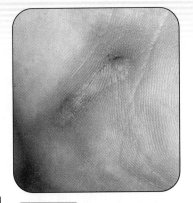

Figure 5-7   Infected wound.

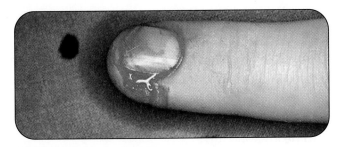

Figure 5-8   Nail avulsion.

Fingernail Injuries

A nail avulsion occurs when a fingernail or toenail is partially torn away from the nailbed (▲ **Figure 5-8**).

Apply an adhesive bandage coated with an antibiotic ointment to the finger and secure the damaged nail in place. A new nail will begin growing to replace the damaged nail in about 1 month. It takes approximately 4 months for a fingernail and 6 months for the nail on the great toe to regrow completely.

A child who catches a finger in a closing drawer or door or who receives a direct blow to the tip of a finger might have bleeding under the fingernail. This causes pressure and can be quite painful. A health care provider should be notified to relieve the pain by making a hole in the surface of the nail.

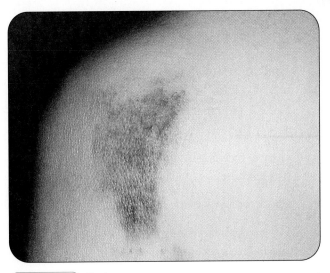

Figure 5-9   Bruise.

Impaled Objects

To care for an impaled object, expose the area. Remove any clothing surrounding the wound. Do not remove or move an impaled object. Stabilize the object by placing bulky dressings or clean cloths around the object.

Splinters

Most splinters are minor nuisances. If a splinter is protruding above the skin surface, remove it by grasping one end with a pair of clean tweezers and pulling. Do not use a needle to dig out a splinter. A deeper splinter will work itself out in several days. To reduce injuries from splinters, check all wooden playground equipment and climbing structures several times a year for areas that are splintering and have them sanded promptly.

Internal Bleeding

Internal bleeding occurs when blood vessels inside the body are broken but the skin doesn't break—a closed wound. A bruise is an example of minor internal bleeding (▲ **Figure 5-9**). Severe internal bleeding can result from a blunt abdominal injury forceful enough to damage large vessels or organs deep inside the abdomen, such as a blow from a baseball bat. It can also result from an injury that breaks a bone and punctures an internal structure, such as a broken rib puncturing a lung. Internal bleeding can also result from a medical problem such as a ruptured appendix. Severe internal bleeding is life-threatening.

What to Look For

- Bruising, pain, and tenderness

- Vomiting or coughing up blood (serious internal injury)

What to Do

1. Control bleeding by applying cold for up to 20 minutes.

2. Check for a possible broken bone.

3. Elevate the injured area to help decrease pain and reduce swelling.

4. Care for shock if serious injury exists. Send someone to call for emergency medical help.

Shock

Shock is the body's response to a disruption somewhere in the circulatory system that prevents blood from circulating in adequate amounts to all parts of the body, especially to the vital organs. Damage to the heart or blood vessels or a decrease in the amount of blood flow can cause shock.

The most common cause of shock in children is from blood loss from either an obvious external wound or from a bleeding wound hidden deep inside the body. Shock can be life-threatening and occurs in the types of injuries sustained in a serious motor vehicle accident, bicycle accident, or fall.

Some degree of shock occurs with all injuries. With minor injuries, the body is able to recover on its own. With more serious injuries, the body cannot recover on its own, and death can result if emergency medical care is not provided.

Shock is most likely to occur within the first few minutes, but it can appear up to several hours after an injury. Treating for shock, whether or not signs and symptoms are present, is the safest way to proceed when caring for a child who has a serious injury. A first aider can slow the progress of shock and even prevent it from occurring by taking the correct steps immediately.

What to Look For

- Pale, cool, moist skin

- Rapid, weak pulse

- Rapid, shallow breathing

- Feeling faint

- Thirst

What to Do

1. Check the ABCs, and use direct pressure, elevation, and pressure points to control any severe bleeding.

2. Send someone to call for emergency medical help.

3. Place the child in the shock position by laying the child flat on the back and raise the feet 8" to 12". This helps to increase the flow of blood to the heart and brain (▼ Figure 5-10). If the child becomes unconscious or begins to vomit, place the child on the side (recovery position).

4. Prevent heat loss by putting blankets or coats under and over the child.

Caution:

DO NOT give anything to eat or drink.

DO NOT raise the legs of a child with a suspected spine injury.

DO NOT raise the legs of a child with a head injury or with breathing difficulties.

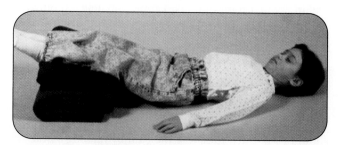

Figure 5-10 Positioning the shock victim.

SHOCK

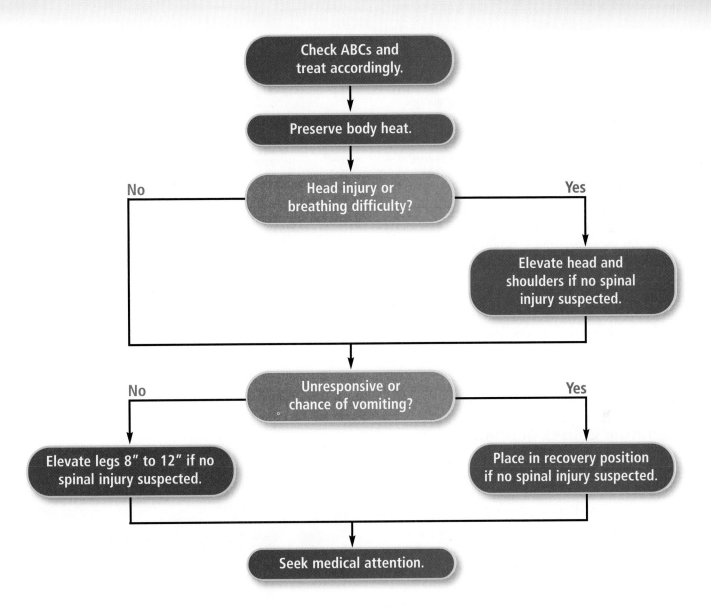

Anaphylaxis

Children who have allergies to such common agents as pollen, molds, dust, animal dander, or certain foods learn that avoidance is the best way to prevent the unpleasant reaction that their bodies produce. Most common allergic reactions can be brought under control by removing the cause from the child's environment or diet.

An uncommon and far more serious allergic reaction is known as anaphylaxis, which is a type of shock that can be fatal if not reversed within minutes. It occurs suddenly, usually within seconds or minutes after coming in contact with the allergen. It causes many allergic symptoms, the most dangerous of which is swelling of the airway that cuts off the child's ability to breathe. If epinephrine, the medication that counteracts anaphylaxis, is not available, death can occur within minutes.

Children who have had an extreme reaction to a specific allergen should have an allergic emergency kit (also known as an anaphylaxis kit or insect sting kit) containing the epinephrine injection. It should be stored with the first aid supplies in the child care center at room temperature. This is not a routine item in all first aid kits; it is a prescription drug intended specifically for the allergic child in an emergency. It contains an easy-to-use mechanism that administers the correct dose of the drug. At least one staff member in a child care center should be taught how to use the kit. A school-aged child who has been given a kit by a pediatrician should always carry it.

Common Causes of Anaphylaxis

Anaphylaxis is unexpected because, initially, neither the child nor parent is aware of the child's extreme allergy to a substance that is harmless to most people. Anaphylaxis can occur in a child who receives a dose of a medication, such as penicillin or tetanus antitoxin, or after eating a food, such as shellfish, nuts, or eggs. A child might also eat a prepared food without knowing that it contains a food additive or ingredient to which the child is highly allergic. Stings from an insect of the Hymenoptera order, which includes bees, wasps, hornets, yellow jackets, and ants, can also cause anaphylaxis. This allergy can develop at any time in life, no matter how many nonallergic stings a child has already had.

What to Look For

- Swelling of the face, lips, and throat

- Wheezing/shortness of breath

- Tightness in the chest

- Dizziness

- Blue/gray color around lips

- Nausea and vomiting

What to Do

1. Check ABCs

2. Send someone to call for emergency medical help.

3. Place an unresponsive child on the side (recovery position). Place a conscious child who is having trouble breathing in a sitting position to make breathing easier.

4. Administer epinephrine immediately. Epinephrine can be given by a parent or a child care provider who has been shown how to administer the medication. More than 1 dose of epinephrine may be necessary to reverse anaphylaxis (▼ **Figure 5-11**).

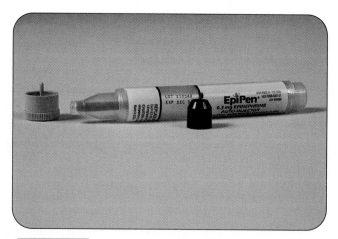

(**Figures 5-11**) Allergic emergency kit.

ANAPHYLAXIS

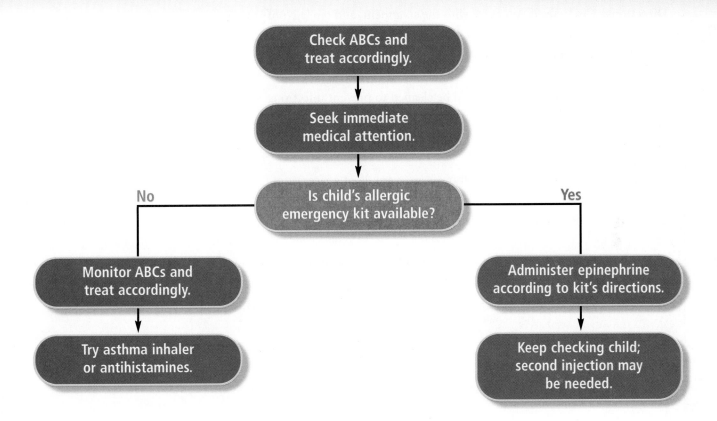

Learning Activities

Bleeding and Shock

Directions: Circle Yes if you agree with the statement, and circle No if you disagree.

Yes No   **1.** Dressing and bandages should be changed if they become wet or dirty.

Yes No   **2.** Minor wounds should be cleaned to prevent infection.

Yes No   **3.** Wounds are sutured to reduce infection and scarring.

Yes No   **4.** A skinned knee or elbow is an example of a laceration.

Yes No   **5.** Puncture wounds often need suturing.

Yes No   **6.** 1 dose of tetanus vaccine provides immunization for a lifetime.

Yes No   **7.** A wound can be sutured for up to 24 hours after the injury.

Yes No   **8.** A first aider should wear disposable gloves when caring for a bleeding wound.

Yes No   **9.** Remove the original dressing if it has become soaked with blood.

Yes No **10.** Shock results when vital organs do not receive sufficient blood.

Yes No **11.** When a child experiences hypovolemic shock, the skin is flushed.

Yes No **12.** A child experiencing anaphylaxis needs sugar immediately.

Yes No **13.** To control severe bleeding, place firm, direct pressure on the wound.

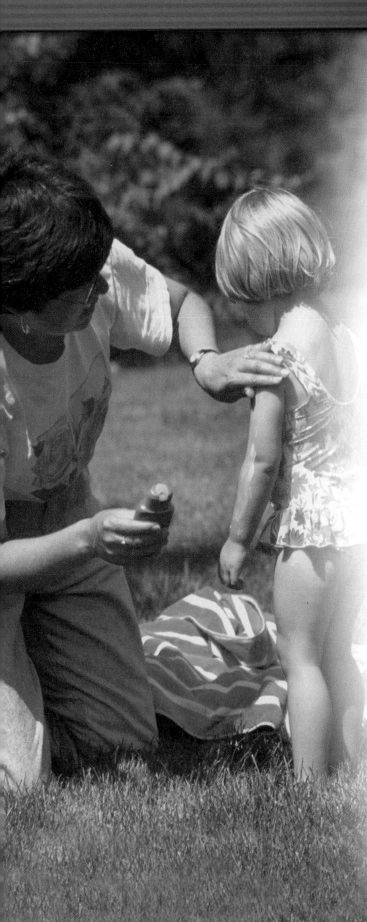

Chapter 6

Burns

Burn Injuries

A serious burn injury can leave a child with long-term physical and emotional scars. Curious children climb and grab; they do not have a clear understanding of what is dangerous; and they are fascinated by fire. Between 50% and 90% of all burns to children under the age of 4 years can be prevented! Most burns to toddlers and preschoolers are scald injuries caused by hot liquids and grease. Flame burns more commonly occur to children 5 to 12 years of age.

Many burn injuries can be prevented if you make burn-proofing a part of child-proofing your home or center. Do you always place hot coffee out of a child's reach? Are your matches always returned to a safe, hidden location? Are you teaching the children in your care that fire is a tool, not a toy?

The skin is sensitive to heat. Temperatures below 111°F generally do not damage the skin. Temperatures above 111°F cause tissue damage, and temperatures above 123°F destroy skin within seconds. Some states have a policy on water temperature limits in a child-care setting. Know your state's policy.

Preventing Burn Injuries

Following basic guidelines for your home or center can greatly reduce the chance of burn injuries.

In the Bathroom

To prevent burn injuries in the bathroom:

- Set the water heater to 120°F.
- When filling the tub, run the hot and cold water together. Turn off the hot water first, so the faucet becomes cool.
- Supervise toddlers and young children in the bathtub so that they do not turn on the hot water.
- Mark the hot water faucet with red fingernail polish or paint to identify it.

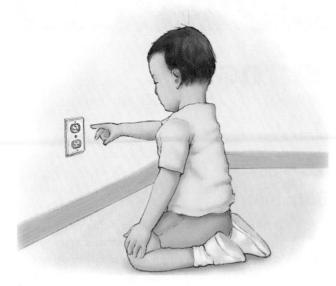

Figure 6-1 Make sure outlets have plastic covers.

In the Bedroom

To prevent burn injuries in the bedroom:

- Keep cribs a safe distance from radiators and electrical outlets.

- Do not use extension cords in a child's bedroom. Position lamps and other electrical appliances in front of wall outlets.

- Cover unused outlets with plastic covers ▲ **Figure 6-1**.

- Do not use a space heater in a child's bedroom.

Electrical Appliances

To prevent burn injuries from electrical appliances:

- Use only electrical appliances approved by Underwriters Laboratory (UL).

- Keep all kitchen appliances at the back of the counter and unplugged when not in use.

- Keep electrical appliances away from water.

- Do not allow electrical cords to dangle over the countertop edge. Regularly check for frayed or damaged electrical cords.

- Do not use extension cords around infants and toddlers. A child can be electrocuted by biting through a live electric cord.

- Do not run electric cords under rugs in areas of heavy traffic.

- Never leave a hot iron unattended.

> **Did You Know?**
>
> More than 27,000 children are hospitalized each year with burn injuries. An estimated 400,000 more are treated in emergency rooms, physicians' offices, and clinics. More than half of all childhood burns occur to children under 4 years of age.

In the Kitchen

To prevent burn injuries in the kitchen:

- Cook on back burners whenever possible. On front burners, turn pan handles in to the center of the stove.

- Remove stove knobs when they are not in use.

- Teach children the meaning of "hot."

- Test foods and formula warmed in a microwave oven. Microwave ovens can warm foods unevenly, creating hot spots.

- Supervise children when they cook.

- Do not store foods that children like to get for themselves, such as cereal, over a stove.

- Do not place hot liquids near the edge of a table or counter.

- Use place mats rather than tablecloths; a child can pull a tablecloth, spilling hot liquids.

- At meals, never pass hot items over a young child's head.

Outdoor Cooking

To prevent burn injuries while cooking outdoors:

- Use only charcoal lighter fluid to light charcoal.

- Never squirt charcoal lighter fluid on a burning fire because it might ignite the entire can.

- Keep the grill away from flammable walls and fences.

- Keep children away from a hot grill.

- Do not throw hot embers on the ground.

Fire Prevention

To prevent fires and to be prepared in the event of a fire:

- Teach children that fire burns.

- Be firm about keeping matches and lighters out of the reach of young children.

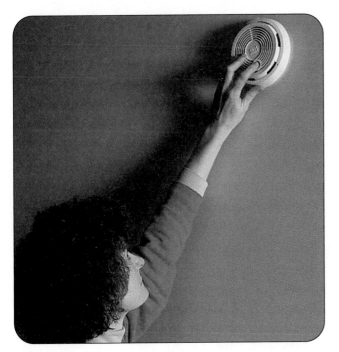

Figure 6-2 Test smoke detectors twice a year.

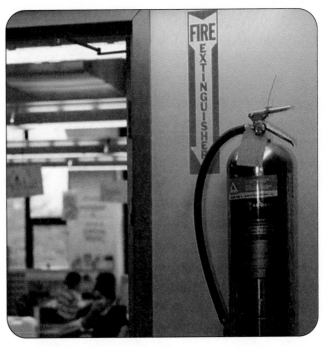

Figure 6-3 Keep fire extinguishers in a highly visible location.

- Do not overload electrical circuits.
- Install smoke detectors and check the batteries in the spring and fall when you change your clocks ▲ **Figure 6-2** .
- Have a fire escape plan with a designated place to meet outside. Hold practice fire drills regularly.
- If you smell gas or suspect a gas leak, open a window or door for fresh air and immediately leave the building. From another building, call the fire department first and then the gas company. Do not turn an electric switch on or off and do not light a match.
- Place barriers around wood stoves and screens in front of fireplaces.
- Make certain that everyone knows where the fire extinguisher is. Do not store a fire extinguisher next to an oven, fireplace, or woodstove where you might not be able to reach it in the event of a fire ▲ **Figure 6-3** .
- Teach children how to call the fire department in your community.

Causes of Burns

Heat burns are the most common burn injury in young children ▼ **Figures 6-4 A-D** . They are caused by contact with flames and other hot sources such as liquids, steam, and appliances.

Chemical burns are caused by corrosive chemicals, which may be stored in garages and basements.

Electrical burns are caused by contact with household current or with lightning.

Ultraviolet rays from the sun burn unprotected skin.

Figures 6-4 A-D Causes of burns.

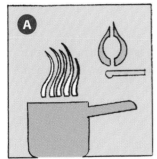

A. Heat.

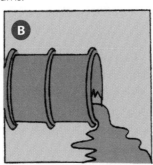

B. Chemical.

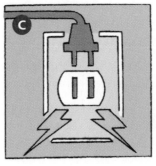

C. Electrical.

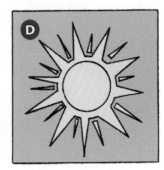

D. Ultraviolet rays.

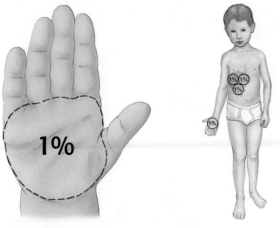

Figure 6-5 The palm of the hand equals 1% of the total surface area of the body.

Figure 6-6

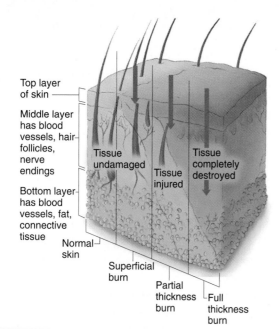

Top layer of skin

Middle layer has blood vessels, hair follicles, nerve endings

Bottom layer has blood vessels, fat, connective tissue

Tissue undamaged

Tissue injured

Tissue completely destroyed

Normal skin

Superficial burn

Partial thickness burn

Full thickness burn

Figure 6-7 Depth of burn injury.

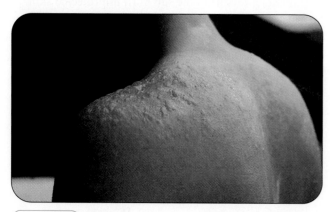

Figure 6-8 Partial-thickness burn: blistered shoulders.

Assessing a Burn Injury

The severity of a burn is determined by three major factors: size, location, and depth. The age of the child and pre-existing medical conditions also influence the seriousness of the injury and the speed of recovery.

The larger the burn, the more serious the injury. Descriptions such as "the size of a quarter" or "half of the back" help to define the size of a burn area. You can estimate the size of a burn on a child by using the child's palm. The palm is 1% of the total body surface, so simply total the palm-sized areas of injured skin (◄ **Figures 6-5 and 6-6**).

Burns can be especially serious when they are located on 1 of the 4 critical areas of the body—the face, the hands, the genitals, and the feet. Unfortunately, children commonly burn these areas when they reach up to stove tops, touch hot appliances, or spill hot liquids in their laps. Flame burns can be especially damaging because the fumes can damage the lining of the airway, causing it to swell and narrow.

A burn is more worrisome in an infant or a young child than in an older child or adult. It is more difficult to correct the imbalance of body fluids caused by a serious burn injury in the younger child.

The depth of a burn is often described as superficial (first-degree), partial-thickness (second-degree), and full-thickness (third-degree). The depth of a burn is determined by the temperature as well as the length of time that the burning substance is in contact with the skin (◄ **Figure 6-7**).

Besides the three factors of size, location, and depth, general health also plays a role in burn severity. Diseases, such as heart or kidney disease, diabetes, asthma, or an immune system disorder, make it difficult for the child with a serious burn to recover and fight off infection.

What to Look For

Superficial (First-degree) Burn. This burn causes minor skin damage.

- Skin pink or red
- Mild swelling, no blisters
- Mild pain

Partial-Thickness (Second-degree) Burn. This burn damages, but does not completely destroy, the full depth of skin (◄ **Figure 6-8**).

- Dark red or bright red skin
- Blisters
- Swelling
- Severe pain

Full-Thickness (Third-degree) Burn. This burn severely damages or destroys the full depth of skin, hair follicles, muscle, nerves, and other tissue.

- Red, raw, ash white, black, leathery, or charred skin

- Swelling

- Little or no pain in area of full-thickness damage because nerves are destroyed. Pain results from surrounding partial thickness and superficial burn areas.

What to Do

1. Stop the burning process.

   - **Heat burns**—Remove the child from the source of heat. If flames are present, smother them by using a blanket or rolling the child on the floor or ground. Prevent the child from running because this fans the flames and helps the fire burn.

   - **Chemical burns**—Brush off any dry chemical that remains on the skin.

   - **Electrical burns**—Be sure the child is no longer connected to the source of the electricity. Turn off the power source before approaching the child.

   - **Ultraviolet burns**—Bring the child indoors.

2. Cool superficial and partial-thickness burns with water.

   - Place the burn in cool water, or cover it with a cold, wet towel if you cannot put it into a container of water, such as with a burn on the face. Rewet the towel every 1 to 2 minutes to keep it cold. This treatment is useful for the first hour after a burn. Do not use forceful running water (▶ **Figure 6-9**).

   - If the burn is caused by a chemical, use running water for 20 minutes to rinse the area. Avoid using a forceful flow, because this can drive the chemical into the skin.

3. Remove surrounding clothing while saturating the burned area. Some synthetic materials melt onto the skin and are difficult to remove. If clothing adheres to the skin, do not try to remove it.

4. Call EMS or contact the child's parent, depending on the extent of the burn injury. See *When to Seek Medical Treatment for a Burn Injury* if you are unsure.

Caution:

DO NOT place ice on a burn, because ice damages the fragile skin that remains.

DO NOT apply burn ointments, petroleum jelly, margarine, or toothpaste to a burn. These products trap the heat.

DO NOT break blisters because they protect the underlying tissue.

When to Seek Medical Treatment for a Burn Injury

If you are unsure of the severity of the burn or the necessity of medical treatment, follow these guidelines. The child should be seen immediately by a health care provider if:

- Burn pain is severe enough that the child is inconsolable and unable to be distracted.

- The child is under 5 years of age and has a partial-thickness burn larger than a quarter.

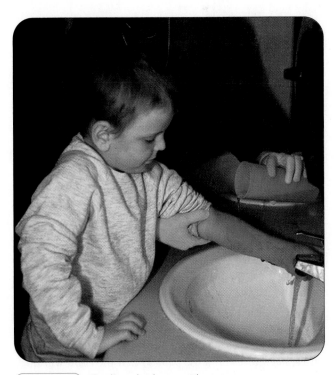

Figure 6-9 Cooling the burn with water.

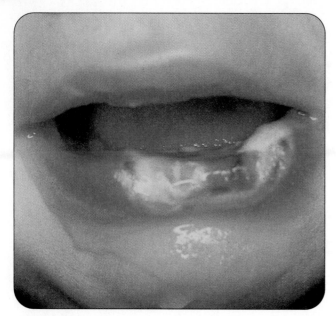

Figure 6-10 Full-thickness electrical burn injury from biting through an electrical cord.

- The child has a full-thickness burn of any size ▲ **Figure 6-10** .

- The child has a pre-existing medical condition.

- The burn is on the child's face, hands, feet, or genitals, or encircles the arm, leg, or chest.

- The burn was caused by a chemical.

- Another injury accompanies the burn.

- The child might have inhaled smoke or flames.

- Signs of abuse are present, such as cigarette burns, a clear border of submersion on a burned extremity, or a burn injury with an explanation that does not seem plausible.

Sunburn Precautions

Unprotected skin is exposed to the harmful ultraviolet rays of the sun whether the day is sunny or cloudy. Repeated exposure to the sun causes early aging of the skin and changes that can allow skin cancers to occur later in life. Skin can be damaged by ultraviolet rays whether it burns or tans, and the harm from repeated unprotected and under-protected exposures is cumulative.

A mild sunburn is usually a superficial burn that is red, painful, and tender. It can worsen as the day progresses, even hours after the child comes inside. A more serious sunburn is a partial-thickness burn characterized by blisters, chills, nausea, and intense pain so that the child will not tolerate clothing on the area. To help relieve the discomfort

of a child's sunburn, use cool water liberally and give a mild analgesic, such as acetaminophen. Over-the-counter sunburn remedies can be applied to non-blistered skin after the first 24 hours. Consult the child's health care provider if the child has any of the symptoms that accompany a more severe burn.

Protecting skin from the sun is essential to avoid sunburn now and to protect against the long-term damage that years of exposure to ultraviolet rays can produce.

- Limit children's exposure to direct sunlight from 11:00 a.m. to 3:00 p.m.

- Use a sunscreen with a sun protection factor (SPF) of at least 30, regardless of the skin's tanning ability. The SPF number indicates the amount of protection the product provides. The higher the number, the greater the protection.

- Choose sunscreens that block both UVA and UVB rays.

- The zinc oxide used in some sunscreens increases the effectiveness of the product and is water resistant.

- Apply the sunscreen liberally to exposed areas such as the face, the back of the neck, the shoulders, behind the knees, and the tops of the feet. Reapply sunscreen often. Products that claim to be water-proof can be washed away in water or by sweating. Do not apply any sunscreen products to a rash or an open cut.

- Apply sunscreen $^1/_2$ hour before going outside.

- The reflection of ultraviolet rays off the water at a pool, lake, or ocean and off the sand at the beach increases the intensity of the sun's rays. In these locations, use cover-ups such as shirts, hats, and an umbrella.

- Children under 1 year of age require special protection. They should have almost no exposure to direct sun and should not be taken to a beach. If exposed to direct sun, they should have all skin covered with clothing and wear a hat. Manufacturers of sunscreens recommend that their products not be used on infants under 6 months of age.

- Some antibiotics can increase a child's sensitivity to the sun's rays. Check medication containers for warning labels.

- Do not tell a child that a tan is a sign of good health or beauty. It is important to educate even young children about the risks of sun exposure to prevent unnecessary sunburns now and sun-related health problems later in life.

THERMAL BURNS

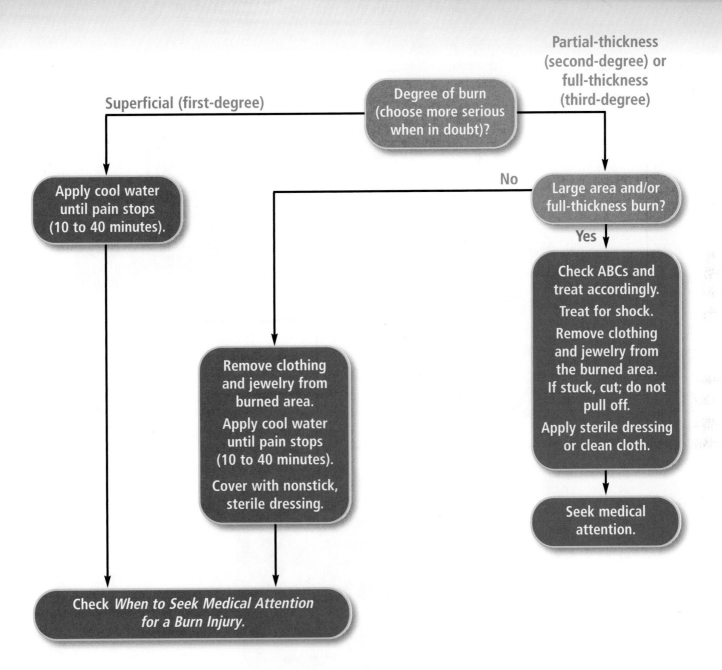

Degree of burn (choose more serious when in doubt)?

Superficial (first-degree) → **Apply cool water until pain stops (10 to 40 minutes).**

Partial-thickness (second-degree) or full-thickness (third-degree) → **Large area and/or full-thickness burn?**

No → **Remove clothing and jewelry from burned area. Apply cool water until pain stops (10 to 40 minutes). Cover with nonstick, sterile dressing.**

Yes → **Check ABCs and treat accordingly. Treat for shock. Remove clothing and jewelry from the burned area. If stuck, cut; do not pull off. Apply sterile dressing or clean cloth.** → **Seek medical attention.**

Check When to Seek Medical Attention for a Burn Injury.

ELECTRICAL BURNS

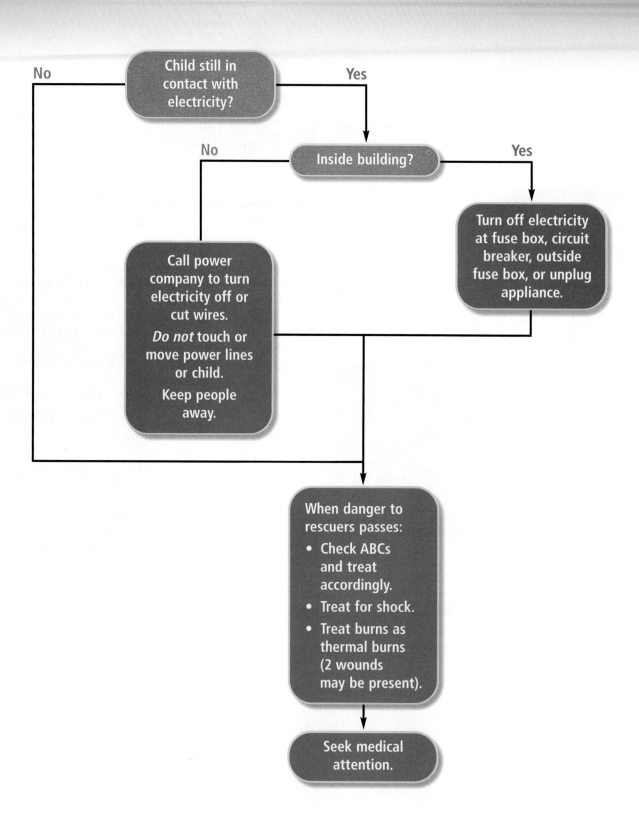

Child still in contact with electricity?

No ────────── Yes

Inside building?

No ────────── Yes

Turn off electricity at fuse box, circuit breaker, outside fuse box, or unplug appliance.

Call power company to turn electricity off or cut wires.

Do not **touch or move power lines or child.**

Keep people away.

When danger to rescuers passes:

• **Check ABCs and treat accordingly.**

• **Treat for shock.**

• **Treat burns as thermal burns (2 wounds may be present).**

Seek medical attention.

What Children Should Know

Children should know where the fire extinguishers are located. Extinguishers should be used only by a trained adult and only if the fire is small and contained.

Children should know the fire escape plan of their child care center. It should be posted in every room and practiced. There should be 2 ways of exiting each room and a place where everyone meets outside. Do not go back inside for any reason.

Children should know to use stairways, not elevators, when leaving a burning building.

Children should know to tie long hair back and not to wear loose-fitting clothes while cooking or standing next to an open flame. Hair and clothing can easily catch on fire.

Children should know that neither they nor their friends should play with matches or lighters. Instruct children to tell a teacher or parent if they find any.

Children should know the phrase, "Stop, drop, and roll." This will remind them to smother flames on their clothing by dropping to the ground and rolling. Running when clothes catch on fire helps the fire burn and increases the chance of inhaling smoke and flames. Also, teach children to cover their faces with both hands when rolling.

Children should know that a fire needs air to burn. Grease fires in a kitchen should be smothered with a lid, not doused with water.

Children should know to crawl to avoid breathing smoke and poisonous fumes when leaving a burning building. The cleanest air is found low to the ground.

Children should know that if they are in a burning building, and come to a closed door, they should feel it with their hands. If the door is hot, there is smoke or fire on the opposite side. Do not open it.

Children should know that if they cannot escape a burning building, they should crawl to a room that has a telephone or a window to the outside. Call the emergency rescue number in your area. Signal for help from the window if there is no fire below that window.

Children should know that they should never go into a closet or under a bed. Rescuers won't be able to find them.

Children should know that the fire safety information they know might save a life.

Children should share what they know with their friends and parents.

What These Children Knew Saved Lives

Cris, age 6, was helping his mother decorate the Christmas tree, when he accidentally leaned back into a table decoration, with candles, and ignited his sweatshirt. Cris had watched the Firebusters program and remembered to "Stop, Drop, and Roll" when your clothes catch fire. He was not injured as a result of his actions.

5-year-old Abby, asleep in the mobile home of the grandparents she and her cousin were visiting, awoke at 1:00 a.m. to find fire and smoke in her room. Frightened as she was, Abby remembered the Learn Not to Burn presentation at her school a few months earlier. Abby dropped to the floor and crawled the length of the 65-foot home to awaken her grandparents and cousin. All four escaped unharmed, although the home was completely destroyed.

Kate, age 8, responded successfully to an early morning fire in her home. The fire had cracked windows with its heat, setting off the burglar alarm. Hearing this, Kate woke up coughing to a home filled with smoke. Her bedroom door was closed. Kate reacted quickly. Crawling on her hands and knees, she moved over to the door and felt the knob. It was hot. Kate then crawled back to her sleeping sister and woke her up. After breaking the window with a rocking chair, as her father had taught

her in their home escape planning, Kate made sure her sister was safely outside before leaving the burning house herself.

Marcus, age 9, was in the bathtub when he heard his 6-year-old brother yelling. Jumping from the tub, he discovered that the younger brother had set his clothing on fire while playing with a lighter. Marcus first threw his towel at him. Realizing that this was not extinguishing the flames, he ordered his brother to "Stop, Drop, and Roll." The local fire department had presented 2 fire safety programs at Marcus's school in the previous 6 months.

Celelana's family's 3-story apartment house was the target of an incendiary fire. When a smoke detector alerted her mother to the danger, she instructed her daughter to get out quickly. 6-year-old Celelana located her 4-year-old sister, crying in her bedroom from fear of the smoke, and pulled her to the floor. She told the younger girl, "We must crawl under the smoke to get out." Their mother found them both sitting on the grass in the front of the house, which was by then engulfed in flames. Celelana told her she had learned the steps she followed from "Fireman Friendly" at her school.

Source: National Fire Protection Association, Quincy, Mass.

Learning Activities

Burns

Directions: Circle Yes if you agree with the statement, and circle No if you disagree.

Yes   No   **1.** Some states have a policy on water temperature limits in a child care setting.

Yes   No   **2.** Apply burn ointment, petroleum jelly or butter to soothe burned skin.

Yes   No   **3.** For many burn injuries, applying ice can limit the extent of the damage.

Yes   No   **4.** A child should be seen by a health care provider for a full-thickness burn of any size.

Yes   No   **5.** Break blisters that form over a burn to relieve pressure.

Yes   No   **6.** Some antibiotics can increase a child's sensitivity to the sun's rays.

Yes   No   **7.** A child should limit exposure to the sun between 11 a.m. and 3:00 p.m.

Yes   No   **8.** Only children who are susceptible to sunburn need sunscreen.

Chapter 7

Head and Spine Injuries

njuries to the head and spine can be devastating because these injuries can affect a person's ability to make decisions, communicate ideas, and control body movement. With the passage of time, wounds, burns, and broken bones will heal. But the same cannot always be said of head and spine injuries. Some injuries to the brain and major nerves of the spine result in damage so severe that function cannot be restored no matter how much time and medical care is devoted to recovery.

Head Injuries

Head injuries are common during the childhood years. Most are superficial, with bruising and swelling of the skin such as a "goose egg," but some can be severe enough to cause permanent brain damage or even death. The Centers for Disease Control estimates that falls account for more than half of all head injuries to children under 5 years of age. In children older than 5 years of age, head injuries are caused equally by sports, falls, and motor vehicle accidents.

Head injuries are so common in young children in part because a child's head represents a larger percentage of both body size and body weight than an adult's head. A newborn's head is a full one quarter of the total body mass. Child care providers who care for young infants are aware that an infant's neck muscles have difficulty controlling the movement of their disproportionately heavy heads **Figures 7-1 and 7-2 ▶**.

Did You Know?

+ Almost 30% of all childhood injury deaths result from head injuries.

+ Each year, an estimated 29,000 children suffer permanent disability from moderate or severe head injury.

Centers for Disease Control: Childhood Injuries in the United States.

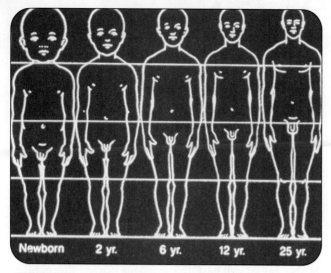

Figure 7-1 A young child's head is proportionately larger than an adults head.

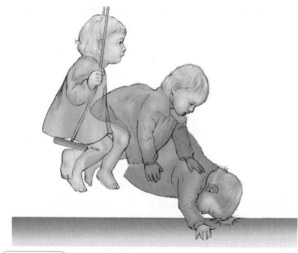

Figure 7-2 A young child's heavy head is the first point of impact in a fall.

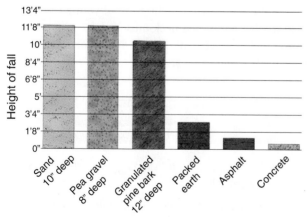

Figure 7-3 This graph shows the approximate height from which a falling child would sustain internal head injury on each playground surface. Source: Franklin Research Center, Norristown, Pa.

The larger, heavy head remains an issue for toddlers and preschoolers, too. When these active children engage in physical play and fall, the head spills forward and breaks the fall against the ground. This situation remains an issue for young children even into elementary school years (◀ **Figure 7-3**).

Bump on the Head

During the first few years of life, when young children are learning to crawl, climb, and walk, small bumps on the head are an everyday occurrence. Because there is little soft tissue surrounding the skull to absorb the blood and other fluids from such injuries, blood collects under the skin in one bulging area often referred to as a "goose egg." Apply ice or a cold pack wrapped in a wet cloth to control swelling.

Scalp Wound

The head has a rich supply of blood vessels so that even minor wounds tend to bleed heavily. However, because of this, cuts on the head rarely become infected.

What to Do

1. Control bleeding. Wear disposable gloves and apply gentle direct pressure to the wound. Bleeding should stop in 5 to 10 minutes.

2. Apply ice or a cold pack wrapped in a wet cloth to control swelling.

3. Clean a minor scalp wound with soap and water and determine the need for stitches. See *About Stitches* in Chapter 5.

Internal Head Injury

Internal head injury refers to damage to the brain. When the head receives a forceful blow, the brain strikes the inside of the skull, resulting in some degree of injury. In addition, blood and other fluids accumulate inside the skull and put pressure on the brain.

Concussion is a term that generally refers to the symptoms of dizziness, nausea, and a loss of consciousness after a violent jarring of the brain. Unconsciousness can last for just a few seconds or for as long as several days.

Because internal head injury can be present even in the absence of a visible skull wound, the following signs and symptoms are the most reliable indicators of internal head injury.

What to Look For

- Loss of consciousness—A child might appear stunned for several seconds after a head injury, but this is not the same as being unconscious.

- Confusion or memory loss—A child can be upset after a head injury but should know where he or she is and what happened.

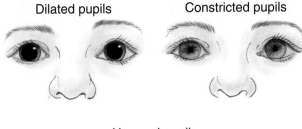

Dilated pupils   Constricted pupils

Unequal pupils

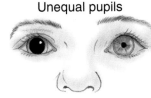

Figure 7-4 Check child's pupils.

- Pale, sweaty appearance
- Severe headache lasting several hours
- Nausea and vomiting
- Blurred vision
- Unusual sleepiness
- Agitation or combativeness
- Pupils of unequal size—The small, black, round centers of the child's eyes should be of equal size and become smaller when exposed to light
  ▲ **Figure 7-4** .
- Difficulty with walking, talking, or balance
- Seizure
- Skull depression—A depressed skull fracture is most often seen in infants.
- Swelling of an infant's soft spot, the fontanel, located on the top of the head
- Fluid dripping from the nose or ear(s)

Cold Pack Alternatives

1. Crushed ice in a plastic bag.
2. Wet washcloth placed in a plastic bag and kept in the refrigerator.
3. Commercial "snap pack" ice packs.
4. Frozen vegetables and other frozen foods.
5. Popsicles for an injury inside the mouth.

Never place cold packs directly against a child's skin. Always wrap the cold pack in a thin cloth to protect the skin.

What to Do

1. Check for responsiveness. Check ABCs and treat accordingly. A child who loses consciousness after a violent head injury should be treated as if he or she has a spine injury. See *Spine Injuries* in this chapter.
2. If child is alert, raise the head and shoulders.
3. For a wound, apply gentle pressure to control bleeding. See *Scalp Wound* in this chapter.
4. Apply ice or a cold pack to control swelling.
5. Observe the child for signs and symptoms of an internal head injury for 24 to 48 hours.
6. Contact EMS and the child's parent immediately if the child shows any signs or symptoms of internal head injury.

Caution:

DO NOT give the child anything to eat or drink.

DO NOT give the child any pain medication.

A child who does not lose consciousness after hitting the head and who quickly returns to normal activity is probably fine. If you are uncertain of the child's condition, contact the parent and have the child seen by a health care provider.

Infants and Head Injuries

An infant's skull has fontanels, also called "soft spots," where the bones have not yet grown together   Figure 7-5 ▶ . Infants are especially vulnerable to head injuries because the skull bones are fragile and the brain is not protected in the area of the fontanels. Therefore, a blow to the head of an infant should always be examined by a health care provider even if, initially, there are no signs of internal injury.

Sleeping after a Head Injury

A child who has had a head injury may be allowed to sleep if it is the normal naptime or bedtime. However, do not allow a child to sleep for longer than 2 hours without being awakened. The child should be easily arousable. Sleeping does not worsen the child's condition. The concern is that a sleeping child cannot be observed for changes in behavior and level of consciousness.

HEAD INJURIES

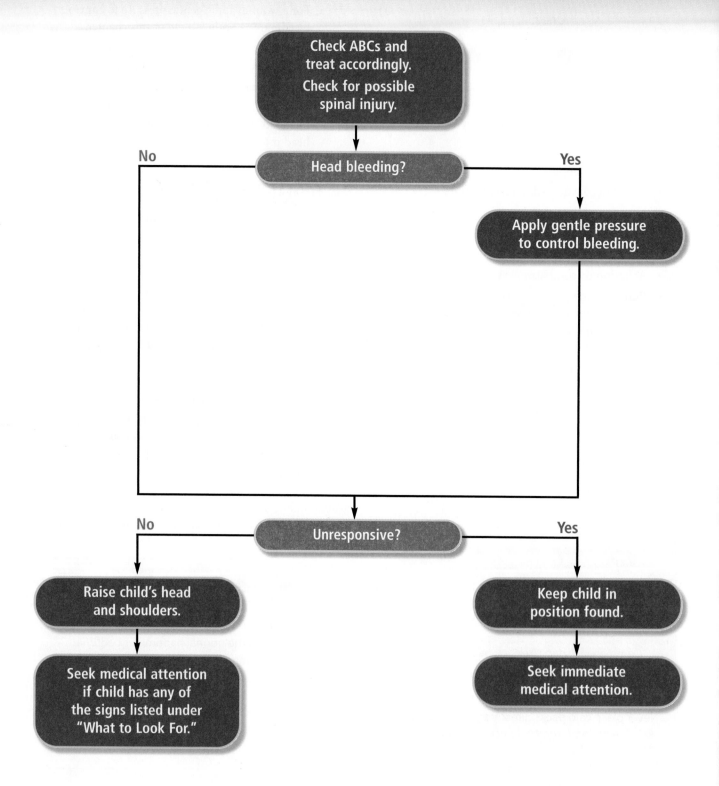

Check ABCs and treat accordingly. Check for possible spinal injury.

Head bleeding?

No

Yes

Apply gentle pressure to control bleeding.

Unresponsive?

No

Yes

Raise child's head and shoulders.

Keep child in position found.

Seek medical attention if child has any of the signs listed under "What to Look For."

Seek immediate medical attention.

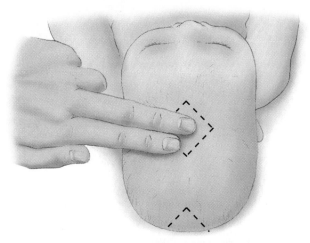

Figure 7-5 Location of infant fontanels (soft spots).

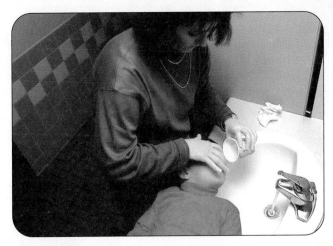

Figure 7-6 Flush a chemical from an eye with warm water.

Eye Injuries

Chemical Injury to the Eye

Chemicals get into children's eyes most commonly from products in spray bottles, such as household cleaners and pesticides. A chemical burn to the eye requires immediate first aid treatment to prevent damage to the cornea, the transparent outer covering of the eyeball. Eye damage can occur swiftly—in less than 5 minutes. An eye that appears only slightly red initially can quickly develop deeper damage, depending on the chemical and the length of exposure.

What to Do

1. Wear disposable gloves and immediately flush the chemical from the eye with warm water. Position the head over a sink with the injured eye down to prevent the rinse water from contaminating the other eye (▲ Figure 7-6). Hold the injured eye open with your fingers and pour water into the eye from an unbreakable cup for 15 minutes. Rinse from the inside of the eye toward the outside. You may need to securely wrap a young child in a large towel to help hold the child still.

2. Call the Poison Control Center to find what further care is needed.

3. Loosely dress and bandage both eyes (▶ Figure 7-7). This will protect the injured eye from unnecessary movement, because both eyes move in unison.

4. Notify the child's parent.

Penetrating Injury to the Eye

Most penetrating eye injuries are obvious. However, you should also suspect a penetrating injury whenever an eye

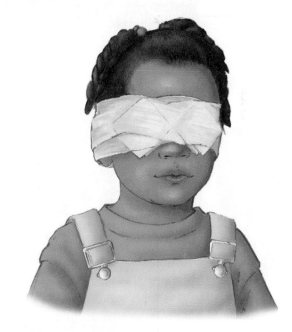

Figure 7-7 Bandaging both eyes.

lid is cut. Do not attempt to remove a foreign object penetrating the eye. Place padding around the object and bandage both eyes. Keep child lying flat on the back. Call EMS. The child should be seen in an emergency medical facility.

Foreign Object in Eye

Eye lashes, dirt, insects, and bits of sand are foreign objects that commonly cause discomfort and tearing of the eyes. If a child has a foreign object in the eye, rubbing the eye can scratch the cornea, the transparent outer covering of the eyeball. A corneal scratch is painful and can introduce infection.

EYE INJURIES

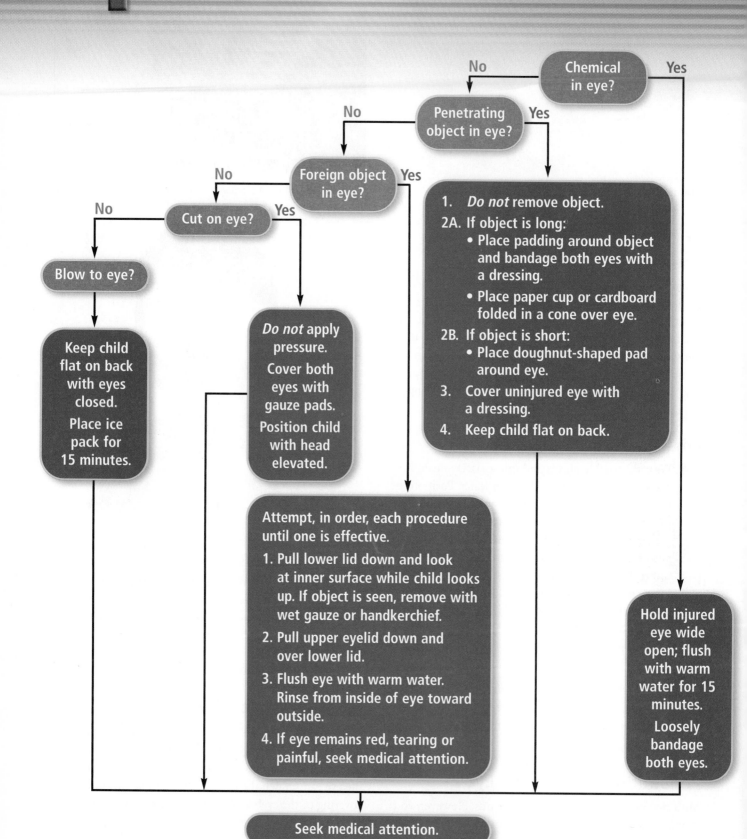

Chemical in eye? — No / Yes

Penetrating object in eye? — No / Yes

Foreign object in eye? — No / Yes

Cut on eye? — No / Yes

Blow to eye?

Blow to eye? → Keep child flat on back with eyes closed. Place ice pack for 15 minutes.

Cut on eye (Yes): *Do not* apply pressure. Cover both eyes with gauze pads. Position child with head elevated.

Penetrating object in eye (Yes):
1. *Do not* remove object.
2A. If object is long:
   - Place padding around object and bandage both eyes with a dressing.
   - Place paper cup or cardboard folded in a cone over eye.
2B. If object is short:
   - Place doughnut-shaped pad around eye.
3. Cover uninjured eye with a dressing.
4. Keep child flat on back.

Foreign object in eye (Yes): Attempt, in order, each procedure until one is effective.
1. Pull lower lid down and look at inner surface while child looks up. If object is seen, remove with wet gauze or handkerchief.
2. Pull upper eyelid down and over lower lid.
3. Flush eye with warm water. Rinse from inside of eye toward outside.
4. If eye remains red, tearing or painful, seek medical attention.

Chemical in eye (Yes): Hold injured eye wide open; flush with warm water for 15 minutes. Loosely bandage both eyes.

Seek medical attention.

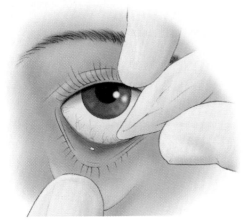

Figure 7-8 Remove a small floating object with the corner of a clean, white cotton handkerchief.

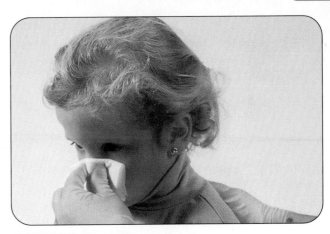

Figure 7-9 Caring for a nosebleed.

What to Do

1. Wear disposable gloves and pull down the child's lower eyelid to look at the inner surface while the child looks up (▲ **Figure 7-8**). A speck of dirt or an insect can usually be removed with the corner of a clean, white cotton handkerchief. If you cannot see the object, it might be under the upper lid.

2. Gently grasp the upper lid and pull it out and down over the lower eyelid. This is often helpful in dislodging the object.

3. If the object remains, flush the eye with warm water. Position the head over a sink, injured eye down. Hold the eye open with your fingers and use an unbreakable cup to rinse from the inside of the eye toward the outside.

4. The child should be examined by a health care provider if the eye continues to be red, tearing, or painful. The foreign body might have scratched the cornea, and this injury can only be confirmed with a special dye and lamp.

Cut on the Eye or Lid

Keep the child in a semi-seated position. Wear disposable gloves. Cover both eyes with a gauze pad and bandage loosely. Do not attempt to flush the eye with water or apply pressure to the injured eyelid. Call the child's parent to have the child seen by a health care provider.

Blow to the Eye

Gently place ice or a cold pack wrapped in a wet cloth around the injured eye for 10 to 15 minutes to control swelling and reduce pain. A black eye or blurred vision might indicate internal eye damage, and the child should be seen by an ophthalmologist as soon as possible.

Nosebleed

Nosebleeds are generally more annoying than serious, especially in a young child. It is the abrupt appearance of a nosebleed that alarms adults. A bump to the nose, crying, laughing, and picking at the nose can all cause a nosebleed. Spontaneous nosebleeds are more common during the colder months, when the air is dry. Bleeding can seem heavier than it actually is. If the child received a direct, forceful blow to the nose, suspect a fracture.

What to Do

1. Wear disposable gloves and pinch together the nostrils on the soft part of the nose below the bridge. Squeeze for 5 to 10 minutes (▲ **Figure 7-9**).

2. Tilt the head forward. Blood is irritating to the stomach and can cause nausea and vomiting.

3. Call the child's parent after 30 to 45 minutes if the bleeding cannot be controlled.

Dental and Mouth Injuries

The following first aid procedures provide temporary relief for dental injuries, but it is important to consult with a dentist as soon as possible.

Knocked-Out Tooth

With proper first aid, a knocked-out tooth can be successfully reimplanted in the socket. It is important to reimplant a baby tooth as well as a permanent tooth, because the baby tooth acts as a space saver for the permanent tooth. A knocked-out or partially knocked-out tooth is considered a dental emergency.

Care after a Nosebleed

+ Encourage the child not to pick the nose.

+ Use a water-based or petroleum jelly to moisten the nostrils.

+ Use a cool mist vaporizer.

DENTAL INJURIES

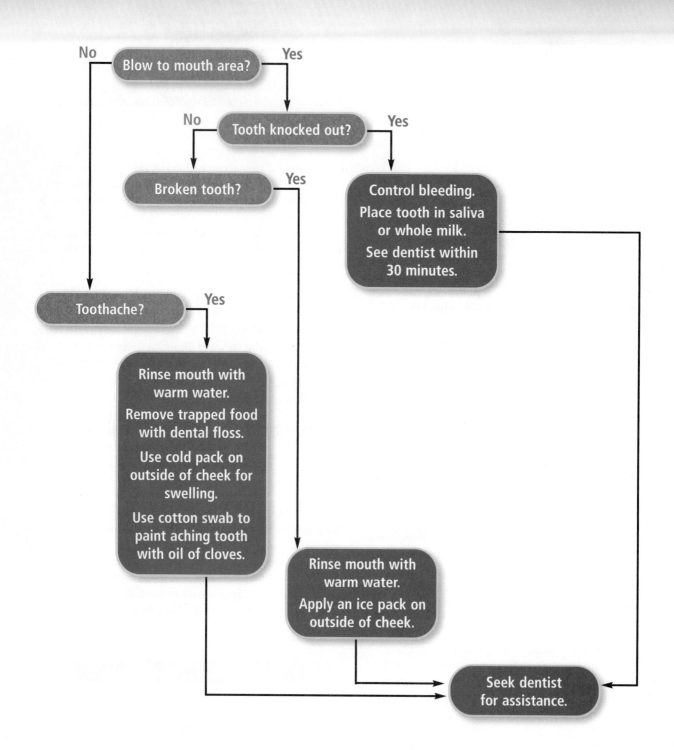

No — Blow to mouth area? — Yes

No — Tooth knocked out? — Yes

Broken tooth? — Yes

Control bleeding.
Place tooth in saliva or whole milk.
See dentist within 30 minutes.

Toothache? — Yes

Rinse mouth with warm water.
Remove trapped food with dental floss.
Use cold pack on outside of cheek for swelling.
Use cotton swab to paint aching tooth with oil of cloves.

Rinse mouth with warm water.
Apply an ice pack on outside of cheek.

Seek dentist for assistance.

What to Do

1. Wear disposable gloves and control any bleeding by placing a rolled gauze pad in the socket.

2. A partially knocked-out tooth should be pushed back into place without rinsing it.

3. A knocked-out tooth should be placed in a container with the child's saliva or whole milk to keep it moist.

4. Seeing a dentist within 30 minutes improves the chances that the tooth will survive.

Caution:

DO NOT clean or touch the root of a knocked-out tooth.

DO NOT allow a young child to hold a knocked-out tooth under the tongue.

Broken Tooth

A child who breaks a tooth should be seen by a dentist as soon as possible (▼ Figure 7-10).

A dentist will file off the sharp edges of a chipped tooth to prevent the tooth from cutting the lip or tongue. If the break extends to the root, the tooth might need more extensive dental work. Have the child rinse with warm water to clean the tooth, and apply ice or a cold pack wrapped in a wet cloth against the face to decrease swelling.

Bite to the Tongue or Lip

A bite to the tongue or lip can be difficult to assess. The mouth has a rich supply of blood vessels and cuts tend to bleed heavily. The amount of bleeding is deceiving, because when blood mixes with saliva, there appears to be more blood than there actually is. Stitches are seldom used when treating cuts of the mouth, unless the wound is large, because the mucous membranes of the tongue and the inside of the mouth are delicate and tear easily.

What to Do

Have the child rinse the mouth with water. Wear disposable gloves and apply pressure with a piece of gauze or a clean cloth to stop the bleeding. Apply ice or a cold pack wrapped in a wet cloth to control the swelling. Call the child's parent and recommend that the child be seen by a health care provider if the cut is deep or extends through the lip border. This cut might need stitches.

Toothache

If a child complains of a toothache, put on disposable gloves and rinse the child's mouth with warm water. Use dental floss to remove any food that might be caught. A cotton ball saturated with oil of clove and placed on the tooth can relieve some discomfort. If pain continues, call the child's parent to recommend that the child be seen by a dentist. See *Teething*, Chapter 17.

Foreign Objects

It should be common practice to keep small objects out of the reach of young children, because of the risk of choking (▼ Figure 7-11).

Be aware that some children put tiny objects, such as beads, buttons, bits of food, plant parts, and pencil-top erasers, in their noses and ears.

Foreign Object In the Ear

You should suspect a foreign body in a child's ear canal if the child pays unusual attention to the ear but does not appear to be in pain. The child might also confide that there is something in the ear. Do not try to remove the object with cotton swabs or tweezers because a young child cannot be relied upon to hold still and the skin of the ear canal is delicate and can be easily damaged. A health care provider can remove the object with special tweezers or a warm water ear flush.

If a child notices that a live insect is in the ear canal, assure the child that the insect cannot travel any farther inside the body. A teaspoon of lukewarm vegetable oil poured into the ear canal kills the insect, but should not be attempted if the child has surgically implanted tubes in the ears. Contact the child's parent and recommend that the child be seen by a health care provider. Never insert a cotton swab or any other object into the ear canal.

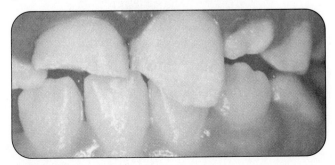

Figure 7-10 Broken teeth. Source: Courtesy of William B. Chan DMD, Tufts University, School of Dental Medicine.

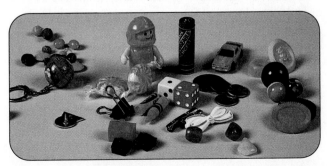

Figure 7-11 Children sometimes swallow tiny objects or put them in their noses or ears.

Foreign Object In the Nose

A foreign object in the nose develops a foul odor and causes a one-sided runny nose within a few hours. The child might pick at the nose if the object is annoying or if it interferes with nasal breathing. It is not unusual for a child to have a foreign object caught in the nose for several days before telling a parent or a child care provider.

The child should try to expel a foreign object by gently blowing the nose if he or she is old enough to have mastered this skill. Otherwise, the child might sniff the object further into the nose. Do not attempt to remove the object yourself with tweezers because this can push the object farther into the nose. The moist environment of the nose allows some objects to expand, making them more difficult to remove. All clinics and health care providers have special tweezers to remove these objects easily.

Swallowed Objects

Except for sharp items, small objects such as buttons and small toy pieces swallowed by a child will pass through the digestive system without complications in 3 to 4 days. A parent might want to call the health care provider if there is any question about the danger of a swallowed object. The local poison control center is also a good source of information. Watch for the swallowed object to appear in the child's stool. Do not give a laxative. Although unusual, if abdominal pain develops during the following few days, the parent should call the child's health care provider.

Spinal Injuries

A spine injury damages the bony column that surrounds and protects the nerves of the spine, known as the spinal cord. These nerves allow sensation and movement throughout the body. Any serious injury to the spinal column and nerves can cause paralysis, or permanent loss of feeling and movement, below the area of the injury.

Spine fractures are becoming increasingly common in children. They most often result from the bending, twisting, or jolting movements that occur with the violent impact of a motor vehicle or bicycle accident or from a sports-related injury. In fact, motor vehicle accidents are the leading cause of spinal cord injury in children under the age of 16, followed by sports-related injuries, acts of violence (almost all from gunshot wounds), and falls. Any child who is unresponsive after an injury should be treated as if he or she has a spine injury.

It is important to know that the nerves inside the spinal column might remain undamaged even if a bone in the spine is fractured. However, if the child is allowed to sit up or is improperly handled, the nerves can become damaged. That is why immobilizing the neck and spine of a child with a suspected spine injury is so important.

What to Look For

- Painful movement of the arms and/or legs; pain can be sharp or radiate down the arm or leg.
- Numbness, tingling, weakness, or a burning sensation in the arms or legs.
- Paralysis of the arms or legs.
- Deformity, or unnatural position, of the child's head and neck.

What to Do

1. If the child is unresponsive, first check for breathing, leaving the child in the position in which he or she was found. Try to determine if the child is breathing by putting your face close to the child's face and listening and feeling for breaths. If the child is not breathing or if you cannot tell, then you must roll the child onto the back as one unit. Use the jaw thrust technique without head tilt to open the airway. See Chapter 3. This is unlikely to aggravate a neck or spine injury. Continue to check the ABCs and treat accordingly.

2. If the child is responsive, immobilize the head, neck and spine, and pad with towels, blankets, or jackets ▼ **Figure 7-12** .

3. If the child begins to vomit, roll the child on to the side (recovery position). If the child is in a dangerous place, gently drag the child to safety, keeping the head, neck, and spine straight.

4. Send someone to call EMS.

Caution:

DO NOT move or change the position of a child with a suspected spine fracture, unless an emergency forces you to do so.

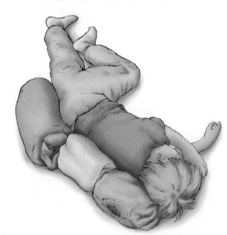

Figure 7-12 Padding the spine of a child with a suspected spine injury.

SPINAL INJURIES

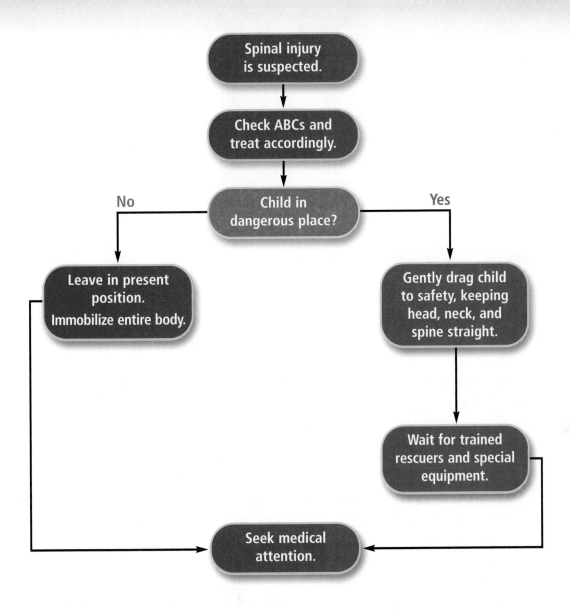

Learning Activities

Head and Spine Injuries

Directions: Circle Yes if you agree with the statement, and circle No if you disagree.

Yes   No   **1.** Head injuries are not as worrisome in infants as in children because infants have fontanels.

Yes   No   **2.** Scalp wounds tend to bleed very little.

Yes   No   **3.** Confusion can be a symptom of internal head injury.

Yes   No   **4.** Pain medication should not be given to a child who complains of a headache after a head injury.

Yes   No   **5.** Rubbing the eye helps to remove a foreign object.

Yes   No   **6.** Rinse an eye by pouring warm water from the outside part of the eye toward the inside.

Yes   No   **7.** Blurred vision after a blow to the eye indicates serious injury.

Yes   No   **8.** Seeing a dentist within 4 to 6 hours improves the chance that a knocked-out tooth will survive.

Yes   No   **9.** Do not move a child with a suspected spinal injury unless the scene is unsafe or child is vomiting and needs to be positioned to keep the airway clear.

Yes   No   **10.** A child who is found unresponsive after a violent injury must be treated as if a spinal injury has occurred.

Yes   No   **11.** It is possible to have a spinal fracture without damaging the spinal cord.

Yes   No   **12.** Diving accidents are the leading cause of spinal cord injury to children under the age of 16.

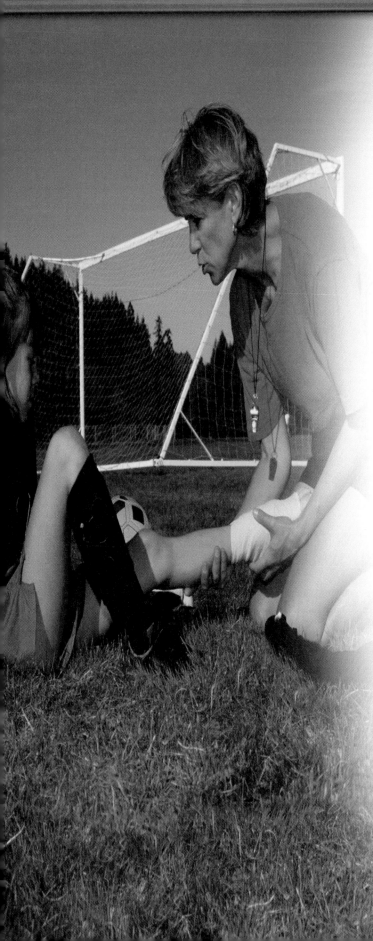

Chapter 8

Bone, Joint, and Muscle Injuries

The bones and joints of young children have not experienced the years of normal wear and tear that comes with aging and are generally more flexible than those of adults. Because of this flexibility, children rarely strain or tear muscles as adults commonly do while stretching, bending, running, or twisting. But flexibility has its disadvantages. Young children are more prone to dislocation of the joints, especially of the elbow, than are adults. Due to their impulsive behavior, they commonly experience broken bones and soft tissue injuries such as bruises.

Fractures

A fracture is a broken bone. A fracture can be a partial break or a complete break in the bone caused by a twist or a direct blow. Fractures are common in children. They can be of concern if there is damage to the *growth plate*, the area of the bone where growth takes place, because damage in this area can cause irregular growth and shortening of the bone. Fractures can also involve damage to the surrounding muscles, nerves, and blood vessels. Fortunately for children, bone healing after a fracture is more rapid in children than in adults. Bones in children have a more generous blood supply, and the thick and strong outer covering of their bones contains more bone-forming cells than adult bones.

It is not always possible to know with certainty that a bone is broken just by looking at it. This is why an X-ray of a suspected broken bone is always taken to confirm that it is fractured and to provide a more detailed look at the bone.

Types of Fractures

- *Closed (simple) fracture.* The skin is not broken where the bone is fractured.
- *Open (compound) fracture.* There is an open wound over the fracture caused either by the bone's breaking through the skin or by the force of the trauma. The bone is not always visible. Open fractures are more serious than closed fractures, because there is greater blood loss and a chance of infection (Figure 8-1 ▶).

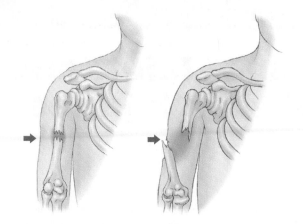

Figure 8-1 Closed fracture (left). Open fracture (right).

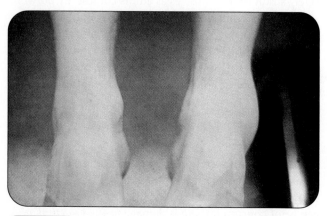

Figure 8-2 Compare injured side to uninjured side.

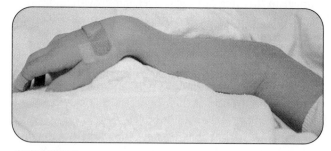

Figure 8-3 Forearm fracture.

What to Look For

- Scene suggests that a serious injury has occurred.
- Pain and tenderness—The child complains of a sharp pain at the injury site.
- Swelling—This is caused by blood and other fluids collecting around the injury.
- Deformity—Sometimes the break in the bone results in an unnatural shape or bend of the body part. Compare the injured body part with the uninjured side to check for deformity (▲ **Figures 8-2 and 8-3**).

- Loss of mobility—The child might be able to move the injured part slightly but will not have full range of motion.

What to Do

1. Remove clothing surrounding the injury. Cut the clothing, if necessary, to avoid moving the injury. Ask the child what happened and where it hurts.
2. Look for DOTS (deformity, open injury, tenderness, swelling).
3. If a wound is present, wear disposable gloves and control bleeding, as necessary. Apply pressure at a pressure point if the bone is protruding through the skin, preventing you from applying direct pressure. Cover the wound with a sterile dressing or large clean cloth to keep it as clean as possible. See the section *Pressure Points* in Chapter 5.
4. Immobilize a suspected fracture by supporting it against the body or by padding the area with towels or pillows in the most comfortable position for the child. This limits movement and pain (**Figure 8-4 ▶**). See the section *About Splinting in a Child Care Center* in this chapter.
5. Apply ice or cold packs wrapped in a thin towel to reduce swelling and pain (**Figure 8-5 ▶**).
6. Elevate an injured arm or leg, as long as it does not cause increased pain. This also helps to reduce swelling and pain.
7. Treat the child for shock.
8. Make arrangements to transport the child to a medical facility.

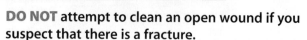

Caution:

DO NOT attempt to clean an open wound if you suspect that there is a fracture.

DO NOT give anything to eat or drink.

About Splinting in a Child Care Center

Knowing how to splint a broken bone can be useful in many situations. However, it is generally recommended that child care providers not splint a young child's broken bone if EMS is available, for several reasons:

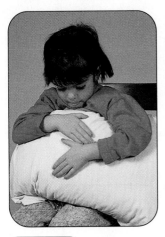

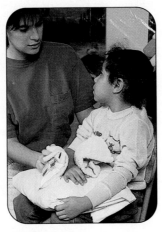

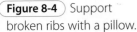 **Figure 8-4** Support broken ribs with a pillow.

Figure 8-5 Place cold packs on both sides of the injured arm.

- A young child in pain cannot be relied on to be cooperative.

- Splints can be applied incorrectly because of the inexperience of the first aider. A splint that is applied too tightly or positions a limb incorrectly can restrict circulation and cause further pain and damage.

- Unnecessary movement of the injury during splinting can cause additional pain and damage to the bone, soft tissue, blood vessels, and nerves.

- The child is often already splinting an injured arm by holding it against his or her chest.

In a child care setting, immobilization of a fracture by padding the injury with towels and pillows is preferred over rigid splinting. Using soft, bulky items provides substantial stability and minimizes movement, so there is less chance of causing additional harm. It is best if emergency medical technicians apply splints. Their knowledge and expertise allow them to apply a splint easily and safely.

Joint Injuries

Dislocations

A dislocation is the separation of a bone from a joint. In children, dislocations commonly happen to fingers and elbows. It takes only a small amount of force to dislocate a child's bone, because children's ligaments are very flexible. A simple quick tug on a child's hand to prevent the child from stepping into the street or to protect against a stumble can be enough to dislocate an elbow (known as *nursemaid's elbow*). Infants and young children should never be picked up by their hands or wrists. Always lift them by placing your hands under their armpits.

What to Look For

- DOTS (Deformity, Open injury, Tenderness, Swelling). A dislocated bone can tear ligaments and damage nerves. Swelling is caused by bleeding within the tissues. Deformity is caused by the unnatural shape of the bone outside of the joint socket. Sometimes the bone will relocate itself immediately, but often it needs to be returned to its proper position by a health care provider. Loss of movement of the joint causes pain if the bone remains dislocated.

What to Do

Care for a possible dislocation in the same manner you would care for a fracture.

Sprains

A sprain is a twisting of a joint, along with a tearing of its supportive muscles and ligaments. Sprains are uncommon in young children because their ligaments are very flexible and stronger than their bones. Often in a traumatic injury, the bone breaks before the ligament is damaged. Sprains begin to occur in children as they progress through grade school, and their joints become more like adult joints.

What to Do

The following first aid measures, known by the acronym RICE (Rest, Ice, Compression, and Elevation), are effective when treating sprains.

1. Rest. Have the child sit or lie down.

2. Ice. Cover the injury with a wet cloth and apply ice or a cold pack for periods of 20 to 30 minutes every 2 to 3 hours for the first 24 to 48 hours. This reduces pain, bleeding, and swelling. Placing a wet cloth directly on the skin transfers the necessary cold more effectively than a dry cloth, yet protects the skin from extreme cold (**Figure 8-6 ▶**). Use an elastic bandage to hold the ice or cold pack in place. Continuous use of ice is not recommended because it can damage the tissue.

3. Compression. Compress the injured area by applying an elastic bandage (**Figure 8-7 ▶**). This limits the collection of blood and other fluids. Start a few inches below and end several inches above the injury. Wrap upward toward the heart in a spiral manner. Use firm, even pressure, making sure you do not wrap too tightly. If the child complains that the fingers or toes are cold, tingling, or becoming numb, loosen the bandage. Remove it only when applying ice.

FRACTURES, DISLOCATIONS, SPRAINS

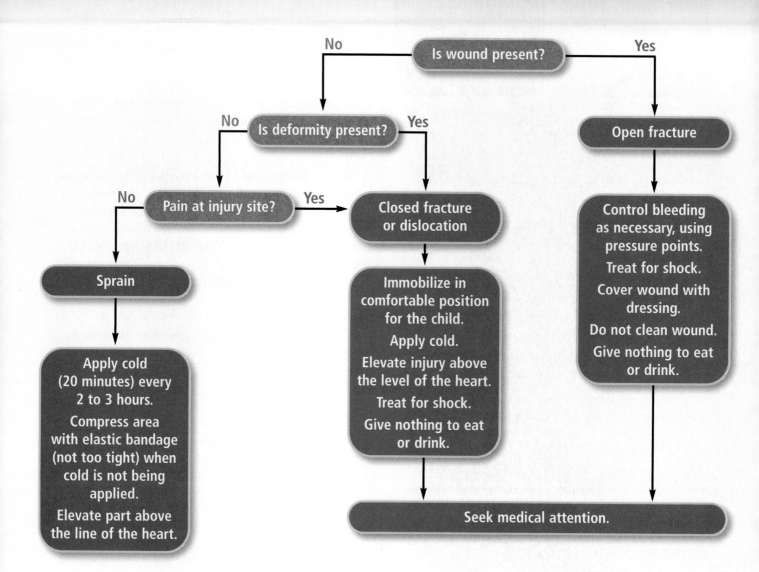

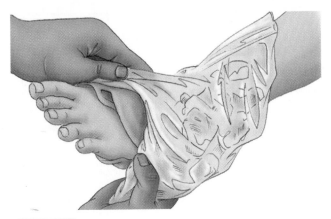

Figure 8-6 Apply ice over a wet cloth.

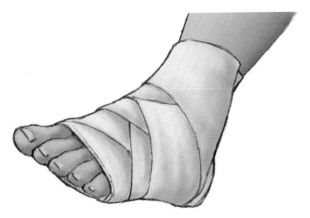

Figure 8-7 Compress the injured area by applying an elastic bandage.

4. Elevation. Elevate the injury above the level of the heart by placing the injured limb on several pillows. This limits blood flow to the injury and reduces swelling.

Caution:

DO NOT wrap a compression bandage too tightly.

DO NOT use ice for longer than 20 to 30 minutes at a time, because it can damage the tissue.

Bruises

Active children, especially those who engage in vigorous play, will often have bruises (contusions). Bruises occur when small blood vessels and other cells break open underneath the skin and bleed into muscles and other soft tissue. Initially, a bruised area is red and swollen; gradually, it turns blue or purple. As the blood is absorbed over the next few days, the area turns yellow and fades as it heals. Apply ice to decrease swelling.

Sports-Related Injuries

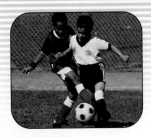

Figure 8-8 Soccer.

Children as young as 4 years of age participate in organized individual and team sports. The pressure from coaches and parents to excel and to win, not just to participate for fun, can be enormous (◄ **Figure 8-8**).

Many injuries can be attributed to repetitive overuse or cross training, which can result in sprains, torn muscles and cartilage, inflamed tendons and joints, and stress fractures.

It is estimated that 4 million children seek treatment in hospital emergency rooms every year as a result of sports-related injuries, and that another 8 million are treated by health care providers for these injuries.

Follow these guidelines to help prevent an injury:

+ The individual who is responsible for coaching a sport should have experience, training, and education in the health risks of training children too vigorously.

+ All coaches, whether paid or volunteer, should be trained in first aid.

+ Children should have a complete physical examination before participating in sports.

+ Children should know what safety equipment is necessary, and it should be available to them consistently. Equipment should fit properly.

+ Playing areas should be free of hazardous debris and regraded when necessary.

+ Time should be included for warm-up and cool-down activities.

+ Pain is an indication that something is wrong. Children should never be told to "work through it."

Adapted from *Sports and Injuries,* The National Youth Sports Foundation for the Prevention of Athletic Injuries, Inc.

Learning Activities

Bone, Joint, and Muscle Injuries

Directions: Circle Yes if you agree with the statement, and circle No if you disagree.

Yes   No   **1.** Fractures in children can result in shortening of the bone.

Yes   No   **2.** Applying heat to a fracture reduces swelling.

Yes   No   **3.** The bone is always visible in an open fracture.

Yes   No   **4.** Positioning an injury above the level of the heart will descrease swelling.

Yes   No   **5.** Clean a wound to check for a fracture.

Yes   No   **6.** Young children are more prone to fractures and dislocations than they are to strains and sprains.

Yes   No   **7.** An elastic bandage should be applied tightly and evenly to control swelling.

Yes   No   **8.** The acronym, DOTS stands for Deformity, Open injury, Tenderness, and Swelling.

Chapter 9

Poisoning

A poison is a substance that, when swallowed, inhaled, absorbed through the skin (as from a plant), or injected (as from an insect sting), can cause illness, damage, and sometimes death. Often, exposure to only a tiny amount can have serious consequences.

Poisoning is one of the most common emergencies in children under 5 years of age. It almost always happens in a home. Swallowed poisons account for most of these emergencies. Fortunately, the incidence of swallowed poisoning has decreased in the last 2 decades because of improved safety packaging. Also, access to regional poison control centers and greater public awareness of poison prevention have helped to reduce accidental poisonings.

However, poisoning still remains a major reason for emergency care and hospital admissions. For every poisoning death among children under 5 years of age, there are 80,000 to 90,000 children who receive emergency medical treatment and 20,000 who need hospitalization. Fortunately, approximately $3/4$ of all poisonings can be successfully treated where they occur.

Swallowed Poisons

Many of the products we use every day to clean our homes, treat our illnesses, maintain our yards, and pursue our hobbies are highly toxic and potentially fatal. They can have tragic consequences when swallowed. In general, the poisonous substances that are the most devastating to children are medications, cleaning products, pesticides, alcoholic beverages, and petroleum products such as gasoline.

Preventing a Swallowed Poisoning

Young children are curious by nature. Colored plastic containers, colorful pills, and never-before-seen items invite the child to explore. Taste is the first sense toddlers and many preschoolers use when investigating something new, regardless of whether it is a toy, food, chemical, or plant. Accidental poisonings often happen when adults

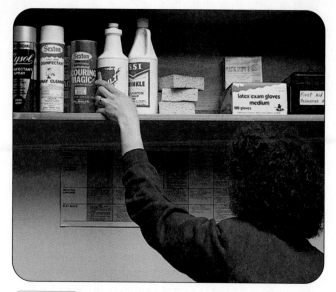

Figure 9-1 Store poisons out of the reach of children.

Some Common Household Poisons

- Acetaminophen
- Alcoholic beverages
- Ammonia
- Aspirin
- Bleach
- Batteries
- Charcoal lighter fluid
- Cleaning products
- Cosmetics
- Drain cleaners
- Gasoline
- Ibuprofen
- Insecticides
- Kerosene
- Mothballs
- Over-the-counter medications
- Toiletries
- Workshop/garage/garden chemicals

are tired or preoccupied, when children have been left alone (even momentarily), and when proper storage or disposal of a poison is either interrupted or forgotten. Most accidental childhood poisonings can be prevented by safe use and proper storage of household products and medicines (▲ **Figure 9-1**).

Safety recommendations for avoiding a swallowed poisoning include:

- Eliminate careless storage of poisons. Keep all chemical substances out of the reach of children, including household products and any chemicals kept in the garage and basement. Store them in locked cabinets or on high shelves. Lock medicine cabinets. Purchase corrosive chemicals such as drain cleaners in single-use quantities whenever possible.

- Conduct a child's eye-level inspection of every room in your child care center or home to see what dangers you can find.

- Avoid interruptions when using a poisonous product.

- Do not store household products with food; the differences between them might not be apparent to a young child.

- Purchase products with child-resistant safety caps whenever possible. Although much safer than standard containers, they are not completely child-proof. Children watch and imitate adult behavior, and some children can master the skill of opening the lids. Also, the lids do not work unless they are completely closed.

- Be careful when storing cosmetics and hair and body care products that do not have child-resistant packaging.

- Keep products in their original, labeled containers. If a poisonous substance is swallowed, correct identification is critical for proper treatment. Do not reuse empty containers such as juice bottles to store chemicals.

- To avoid accidental poisonings with medicines, follow these rules:

  - Keep medicines in a locked cabinet. Never keep medicines on a bedside table or in a drawer.

  - Remember that nonprescription medicines are just as dangerous as prescription medicines.

  - Give prescription medicine only to the child for whom it is intended. What can help one child can harm another.

  - Check the medicine label for the dosage each time you give it. Use a dose-measuring cup or spoon. More is not better when giving medicine.

  - Only one adult in a child care center should administer medicine to avoid an accidental overdose.

  - Never call medicine "candy." This invites a poisoning accident.

  - Flush old medicine down the toilet, and rinse out the container before discarding it.

- Check for poisons when taking a child on a field trip or into a home or other building.

- Keep purses out of the reach of children.

The #1 Poison

In young children, the single most common exposure to a poisonous substance is acetaminophen, a fever reducer and pain reliever. Accidental overdoses occur because parents are not aware that the infant and toddler strengths differ. The infant product is stronger than the toddler product, because it is intended to be given in a small amount from a dropper. If an adult gives the infant liquid to an older child, using a measuring spoon, the child receives too much acetaminophen. In large amounts, acetominophen is toxic. Parents of young children are urged to consult their child's health care provider for the proper dosage and strength.

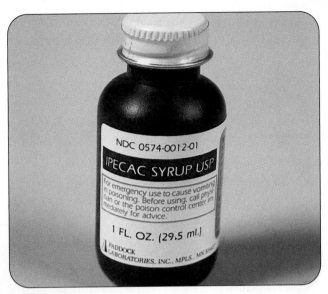

Figure 9-2 Syrup of ipecac.

- Plants can contain potentially dangerous chemicals. These rules apply to plants:

  - Identify all indoor and outdoor plants at your center. Move poisonous plants out of the reach of children.

  - Avoid decorating with the live December holiday plants, including poinsettia, holly, mistletoe, boxwood, and bittersweet. Although festive, all are dangerous and some are extremely poisonous.

  - Outdoors, teach children to keep all plants, including flowers and berries, out of their mouths. Do not share your knowledge of edible wild plants with young children, because they are not always able to identify safe plants correctly when you are not around.

- Be sure that the art product packages in your center are labeled "AP" for approved product or "CP" for certified product. Some art supplies can be toxic if ingested or inhaled.

- Be sure that all lead paint has been removed from your center or home. See the section *Lead Poisoning in Children* in Chapter 17.

Be Prepared

Maintaining good poison prevention habits includes being prepared for a poisoning. Taking the following precautions now will prepare you to respond quickly and appropriately if a poisoning ever occurs in your center or home.

- Keep the telephone number of your local poison control center and EMS posted at every telephone.

- Keep syrup of ipecac in the first aid kit. Ipecac is a plant extract that, when swallowed, is the fastest and most effective way to cause vomiting. It is available without a prescription. Syrup of ipecac is used only to treat swallowed poisons that can be vomited safely; with other swallowed poisons its use can be devastating (▲ **Figure 9-2**). *Never* give it unless the poison control center tells you to do so.

- Keep activated charcoal in the first aid kit, if recommended by your region's poison control center. Activated charcoal is a finely ground powder made from wood that has been exposed to very high temperatures. Activated charcoal works by binding with the poison in the stomach and small intestine and preventing it from being absorbed by the body. It is available without a prescription and is used for treating a variety of poisons, but should only be given if the poison control center tells you to do so.

- Call your local poison control center whenever you have a question about a medicine, household chemical, or plant.

When Poisonings Occur

Poisonings occur throughout the day, but the peak hours for poisoning incidents are between 5:00 p.m. and 9:00 p.m.

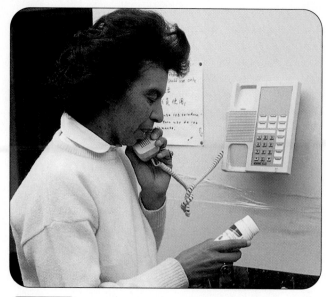

Figure 9-3 If a child swallows a poisonous substance, call your local poison control center immediately.

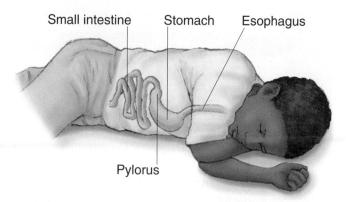

Figure 9-4 The left side-lying position slows the emptying of the stomach.

What to Look For

The signs that the child exhibits depend on the chemical swallowed and the amount of time that has passed. Absorption can begin in minutes, making immediate action necessary. Look for:

- Opened container of medicine or chemical
- Unusual odor from mouth or clothes
- Burns in and around the mouth indicating contact with a corrosive chemical
- Nausea or vomiting
- Abdominal pain or diarrhea
- Drowsiness
- Unconsciousness

What to Do

1. Remove traces of the poison from the child's mouth.
2. Gather information. Remain calm. Try to determine the following:
   - Age and approximate weight of the child
   - What was swallowed
   - Amount swallowed, such as "just a sip," "half of the pills," "all of the liquid"
   - When it was swallowed
   - Child's condition, such as conscious, vomiting, burned mouth, abdominal pain
3. If the child is responsive, call your poison control center (▲ Figure 9-3). Have the child and the poison container with you.

4. Place the child on his or her left side (recovery position). Lying on the left side slows the emptying of the stomach contents. This position also keeps the airway open and allows vomit to drain from the mouth (▲ Figure 9-4).
5. If the child is unresponsive, call 9-1-1 or your local emergency number.
6. Monitor the ABCs and treat accordingly.
7. Call the child's parent.

Caution:

DO NOT give syrup of ipecac to induce vomiting unless told to do so by the poison control center.

DO NOT give syrup of ipecac to induce vomiting if the child is drowsy or unresponsive. The child might choke.

DO NOT give milk or water to dilute a swallowed poison unless told to do so by the poison control center. Milk or water may cause some chemicals to dissolve more quickly.

DO NOT give syrup of ipecac to induce vomiting if burns or blisters are present in and around the mouth.

DO NOT give syrup of ipecac at the same time as activated charcoal. Your poison control center will tell you how and when to use each of these products.

Swallowing any chemical can have serious consequences, but swallowing a corrosive chemical has additional dangers. A corrosive chemical can cause severe burns and pain to the lips, mouth, throat, stomach, and small intestine. Corrosive chemicals should not be vomited because the throat and mouth will be damaged further if exposed to the chemical again. A child who has swallowed a corrosive substance must be treated in an emergency medical facility immediately. This is a life-threatening emergency.

Poison Control Centers: A Life Saver

Poison control centers are the most reliable source of information about poisons. These centers are located throughout the United States and are staffed by experts who have training in toxicology, the study of poisons. They have access to product information on hundreds of thousands of household products and medications. They also have access to information about such uncommon poisons as mushrooms and snake venom. In addition, poison control centers have a variety of informative pamphlets to help you prevent an accidental poisoning.

Poison control centers serve emergency medical facilities, community health care providers, and the general public. They are equipped to answer routine questions and to handle poisoning emergencies. They can determine whether a poisoning can be treated over the telephone or whether the child needs to be seen in an emergency medical facility. If the poisoning can be treated at home, they provide specific directions on what steps to take.

Everyone in the United States can reach a regional poison control center with either a local phone call or a toll-free number. Check your telephone book to obtain the number for the poison control center in your area and post it next to each telephone.

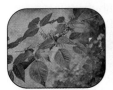
Figure 9-5 A Poison ivy.

Figure 9-5 B Poison oak.

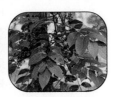
Figure 9-5 C Poison sumac.

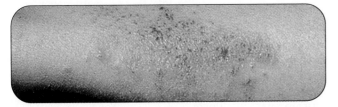
Figure 9-6 Poison ivy rash.

Poisonous Plants

Like many adults, most young children know little about toxic plants and cannot be relied upon to recognize them. Because many young children use their senses of touch and taste when investigating something new, it is not unusual for them to touch and mouth leaves, berries, and flowers. Poisonings can occur from swallowing a plant, absorbing a toxin through the skin, or inhaling fumes from a fire that contains a poisonous plant. Some poisonous plants cause only minor symptoms; some can be deadly. There is no "sure-fire" way to tell a poisonous plant from a nonpoisonous one.

Swallowed Plants

If a child in your care swallows any part of a plant, take the child and a sample of the plant to the telephone and call the poison control center. They will tell you what to do. For the children's safety, learn the names of the plants, trees, and shrubbery around your center.

Poison Ivy, Poison Oak, and Poison Sumac

A small number of plants cause an allergic reaction when they make contact with skin. The best known are poison ivy, poison oak, and poison sumac, all of which are found throughout the United States (▲ Figures 9-5 A-C).

Exposure to the oil of these plants can cause a delayed allergic reaction in the form of a rash that varies in severity. A child can be exposed to the oil of these plants directly by touching the leaves, stems, or roots, or indirectly by touching tools, clothes, pets, or any other article touched by the plant. Smoke from a brush fire containing the burning plant will carry this oil in tiny droplets to the skin and into the nose, throat, and lungs. A reaction can develop from contact with these plants during any season of the year and from handling any part of the plant—not just the leaves (▲ Figure 9-6).

Unfortunately, most people cannot recognize these plants to avoid them. To help everyone avoid them, teach children the short rhyme, "Leaves of three—Let them be!"

What to Look For

Poison ivy, poison oak, and poison sumac rashes can vary from a mild case with itching and redness to a severe case that blisters and swells. Sometimes a severe rash is accompanied by a secondary infection. It commonly takes 1 or 2 days after contact for symptoms to appear.

What to Do

1. If a child in your care is exposed to one of these plants, immediately wash the area with soap and flush with plenty of running water to rinse off the plant oil. Shower rather than bathe. The severity of the rash can be lessened if the soaping and rinsing occurs immediately after exposure.

Poisonous Plants

The following list names some of the more common indoor and outdoor poisonous plants. Though the toxicity varies, ingesting or swallowing any amount of these plants is dangerous.

A
Acorn
Aloe vera
Amaryllis
Anthurium
Arrowhead
Autumn crocus
Avocado leaves
Azalea

B
Baneberry
Belladonna
Bird-of-paradise
Bittersweet
Black locust
Bleeding heart
Boston ivy
Boxwood
Buckeye

Buttercup

C
Caladium
Calla lily
Caper spurge
Carnation
Castor bean
China berry
Chrysanthemum
Crown of thorns
Cyclamen

D
Daffodil bulb
Daisy
Daphne
Delphinium
Dieffenbachia
Dumb cane

E
Elephant ear
English ivy
Eucalyptus

F
Four o'clock
Foxglove

G
Glory lily
Golden chain tree
Ground ivy

H
Holly
Hyacinth
Hydrangea

I
Iris

J
Jack-in-the-pulpit
Jerusalem cherry
Jessamine
Jimson weed (thorn apple)
Juniper

L
Lantana
Larkspur

M
Marijuana
Mistletoe
Morning glory
Mountain laurel
Mushrooms

N
Narcissus
Nightshade

O
Ohio buckeye
Oleander

P
Periwinkle
Philodendron
Pits of apricot, cherry, peach, and plum
Poinsettia
Poison hemlock
Poison ivy
Poison oak
Poison sumac
Privet

R
Rhododendron
Rhubarb leaves
Rubber vine

S
Shamrocks
Skunk cabbage
Sweet pea

T
Tobacco
Tomato leaves
Tulip bulbs

W
Water hemlock
Wisteria

Y
Yew

Nonpoisonous Plants

The following plants are generally considered to be nontoxic. However, it is always possible for an individual to have an allergic reaction from ingesting a part of one of these plants.

A
African violet
Aluminum plant
Asparagus fern

B
Baby's breath or baby's tears
Bachelor buttons
Begonia
Boston fern

C
Cacti (certain varieties)
Christmas cactus
Coleus

Corn plant
Crape myrtle
Creeping Jenny
Crocus

D
Dahlia
Dandelion
Dogwood
Dracaena

E
Easter lily

F
Forget-me-not
Forsythia
Fuschia

G
Gardenia
Geranium
Gloxinia

H
Hibiscus
Honeysuckle
Hoya

I
Impatiens

J
Jade plant

K
Kalanchoe

L
Lipstick plant

M
Monkey plant

N
Norfolk pine

O
Orchid

P
Pansy
Petunia
Phlox
Prayer plant
Purple passion

R
Rose
Rubber plant

S
Sedum
Sensitive plant
Snapdragon
Spider plant
Swedish ivy

T
Tiger lily

U
Umbrella plant
Umbrella tree

V
Venus flytrap
Violet

W
Wandering Jew
Wax plant
Weeping fig
Weeping willow

Y
Yucca

Z
Zebra plant
Zinnia

2. Notify the parent at the end of the day. Most children do not know about their contact until several hours or days later, when the itching and rash begin. If the child has a moderate to severe reaction, a few days at home would be appropriate.

3. A child can return to your center or home when feeling better, as long as the rash is covered with a nonstick dressing. This protects the child's rash from becoming infected. It also prevents others from contact with the weeping blisters even though the fluid in the blisters does not spread the rash. Be certain that all staff know this often-misunderstood fact.

Caution:

DO NOT touch or rub the area if you suspect contact with poison ivy, poison oak, or poison sumac, because you can spread the oil.

Inhaled Poisons

Poisoning by inhalation can occur dramatically, as in smoke inhalation during a building fire. It can also occur insidiously, as in carbon monoxide poisoning from a faulty furnace, a kerosene space heater, or a car motor running in an enclosed garage. Sadly, it can also occur when a child experiments with intentionally inhaling a chemical, such as the fumes from rubber cement and model glue.

Although the flames from a burning building are frightening, it is the smoke and fumes that are the most deadly. Toxins are absorbed, and fumes irritate and burn the airway, causing swelling hours after the exposure.

In other, less dramatic cases of inhaled poisoning, a child might complain of headache, nausea, or vomiting. A building-wide poisoning such as carbon monoxide will affect everyone in the building, including pets. Remove the child from the toxic area. Call EMS, if necessary.

The Carbon Monoxide Problem

Carbon monoxide (CO) is a poisonous gas that is deadly if inhaled in sufficient quantities for enough time. Dangerous concentrations of CO can occur anytime combustion (burning) takes place in a poorly ventilated area.

The biggest problem with CO is that it "sneaks up" on its victims. Carbon monoxide is odorless, tasteless, and invisible, and does not sting or burn the skin or eyes. There is no warning that it is present. Breathing carbon monoxide in a dangerous amount over a short period of time leads to unconsciousness and death. Breathing small amounts of it over a long period of time is equally dangerous, because the effects are cumulative over time.

To minimize the risk of carbon monoxide poisoning, follow these rules:

+ Be sure that the building's central heating system is properly maintained and inspected. Dryers and water heaters powered by gas should also be inspected.

+ Never use a charcoal grill, hibachi, or gas grill inside a building or garage.

+ Never use a gasoline or kerosene space heater in a child care setting.

+ Never use a gas stove or oven to heat living areas.

+ Always check that burners on a gas stove are turned completely off when finished cooking.

+ Never run a car engine in an attached garage, especially with the garage door closed.

+ Install carbon monoxide detectors in the living and sleeping areas of the center. These detectors sound an alarm if the CO level becomes unsafe.

Inhalation Injuries and Older Children

Sometimes older children experiment with inhaling solvents in products such as model glue, white correction fluid, or rubber cement, or they may spray various aerosols from cans directly into the nose in the hopes of "getting high." Although this can be a part of a larger drug addiction problem, it may also be part of the normal inquisitiveness about the forbidden at this age. Inhaling these vapors can cause disorientation and behavior changes.

Repeated abuse can permanently damage the liver and the brain. Elementary school-aged children must be taught that inhaling these vapors is dangerous and that they should avoid participating in this type of recreational activity in their preteen and teenage years.

Learning Activities

Poisoning

Directions: Circle Yes if you agree with the statement, and circle No if you disagree.

Yes   No   **1.** Always induce vomiting with syrup of ipecac in a conscious child who swallows a poison.

Yes   No   **2.** Give several glasses of water or milk to dilute a poison before calling the poison control center.

Yes   No   **3.** Activated charcoal given at the same time of syrup of ipecac improves syrup of ipecac's ability to empty the poison from the stomach.

Yes   No   **4.** There is no reliable way to tell a poisonous plant from a non-poisonous plant.

Yes   No   **5.** Warn others that poison ivy can be spread from contact with open blisters.

Yes   No   **6.** Toxic effects from an inhaled poisoning are almost always apparent immediately.

Yes   No   **7.** Carbon monoxide is an odorless gas.

Yes   No   **8.** If exposed to poison ivy, wash the area immediately with soap and flush with running water.

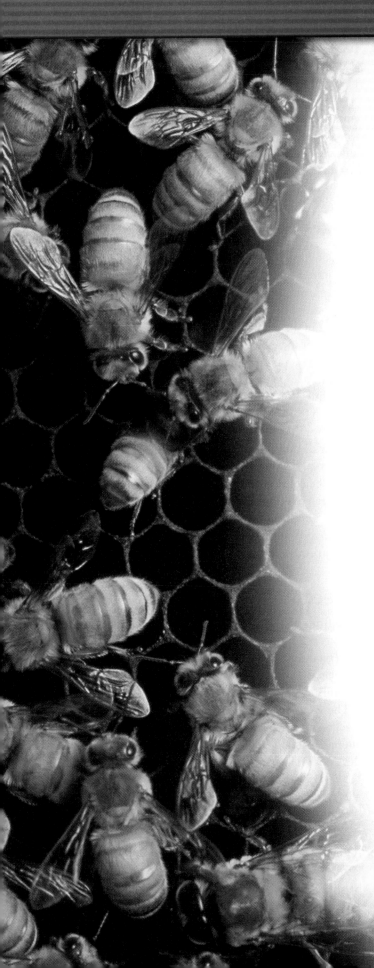

Chapter 10

Bites and Stings

Animal Bites

Dogs are responsible for almost 90% of all animal bites in the United States each year. Their love and loyalty, however, make them one of the most popular pets. They can help a child learn to accept responsibility, understand about caring for others, and build self-confidence. Unfortunately, each year there are nearly 1.5 million serious dog bites; 80% of them involve preschool or school-aged children. The majority of these bites are provoked by children teasing or mistreating the animal.

Cats are less likely to bite than dogs, but cat bites are more likely to become infected. Wild animals such as raccoons, chipmunks, and squirrels also bite. Any bite that breaks the skin can become infected.

The most dangerous infection that can develop after an animal bite is rabies, a viral disease. The rabies virus is present in the saliva of an infected animal and is transmitted to a person through a bite. The disease affects the brain and nervous system. Once rabies symptoms develop, the disease is always fatal. To ensure that this deadly illness does not develop, a person who has been bitten or scratched must be evaluated immediately by a health care provider and, if necessary, receive the rabies vaccine in a series of 5 injections.

Any warm-blooded animal can carry rabies; however, the animals most commonly infected are raccoons, bats, skunks, foxes, and coyotes. According to the Centers for Disease Control, more than 80% of rabies cases in the United States occur in skunks, raccoons, and bats. A bite from a stray cat or dog is also of concern, because these animals probably are not immunized. If a child is bitten by one of the animals more commonly infected with rabies, it must be assumed that the animal is rabid.

Caged animals popular in homes and child care centers, such as hamsters, gerbils, and guinea pigs, are generally healthy and do not carry rabies. This is also true for domestic ferrets. Cold-blooded animals do not carry rabies, although bites from such animals as snakes, spiders, and turtles can become infected.

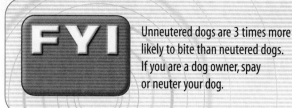

Unneutered dogs are 3 times more likely to bite than neutered dogs. If you are a dog owner, spay or neuter your dog.

Why Do Dogs Bite?

No matter how obedient and loving dogs can be, they are still animals. Dogs are not usually mean or aggressive, but they will react when threatened or upset or when their hunting instinct is triggered. In these situations, dogs may surprise family or strangers with unexpected aggressiveness or biting.

Safety rules about dogs include:

+ Never mistreat, tease, or make threatening gestures toward a dog.

+ Never disturb a dog that is eating or sleeping.

+ Supervise a child feeding a dog.

+ Enter a yard where there is a dog only with the owner accompanying you.

+ Do not attempt to get a dog to chase you.

+ Never make a quick movement around a dog that might startle or frighten the dog.

+ Never break up a dog fight.

+ Avoid strange dogs, especially if the animal is sick or injured.

+ If you are approached by an unfamiliar dog, stop, stand still, and speak softly.

Many animals known to carry rabies are nocturnal. Should you see one of these animals during the day, assume that it is sick. Keep children away from the animal and call the animal control officer in your community. Do not corner or try to capture the animal yourself.

If a child is bitten by a cat or dog, the parent must check with the animal's owner and verify the animal's current immunizations. Pet owners must keep their pet immunizations up-to-date. Animal bites that break the skin, however small, introduce bacteria into the blood. Animal bites that do not break the skin are not serious.

Wear disposable gloves and control bleeding. If the wound is large or might need stitches, do not attempt to wash the wound. Wash a small wound with soap and water. Some bleeding during washing helps to remove bacteria. Apply a clean gauze dressing, if needed.

Identify the animal, if possible, and check the animal's immunizations.

Seek medical attention if the wound is large or needs stitches. For smaller bites that break the skin, call the child's parent. Encourage the parent to contact the child's health care provider.

Human Bites

Biting occasionally occurs among young children who have not yet learned socially acceptable behavior for expressing themselves and meeting their needs. Fortunately, the urge to bite usually disappears on its own in the course of preschool development.

Many of these bites are minor and more of an emotional upset than a physical injury. However, the human mouth contains a large number of bacteria, some of which can cause infection through a bite. In fact, the likelihood of infection from a human bite is greater than from an animal bite. Bites that do not break the skin are not serious.

Wear disposable gloves, and wash the wound with soap and water. Notify the child's parent if a bite breaks the skin. The child might need a tetanus shot or antibiotics.

Repeated biting is unacceptable behavior in a child care center. This behavior should be dealt with promptly to discourage the child from repeated incidents of biting and to protect the other children from injury.

Insect Stings

Bites from such insects as mosquitoes, gnats, fleas, and flies seldom require any medical attention. However, stings from the *Hymenoptera* order of insects, which includes bees, hornets, yellow jackets, wasps, mud daubers, and ants, are painful and can even be deadly (**Figures 10-1, 10-2, 10-3 ▶**).

These insects inject venom that produces a mild local reaction and, in a small percentage of people, a more severe allergic reaction. A little less than 1% of the population develops an allergy to this venom, and it is estimated that between 50 and 100 people die every year from a severe allergic reaction to *Hymenoptera* venom.

What to Look For

A normal reaction to an insect sting is a painful surprise but is not serious. It lasts up to a few hours and is characterized by stinging pain, redness, and mild swelling. Sometimes

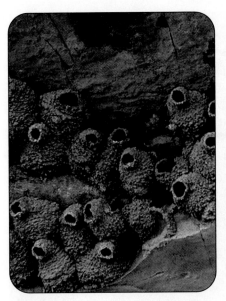

Figure 10-1 Mud dauber nest.

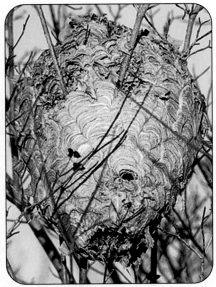

Figure 10-2 Hornet and yellow jacket nest.

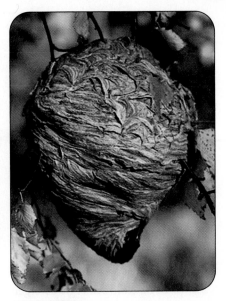

Figure 10-3 Wasp nest.

pain and swelling can last a few days. However, these normal reactions are not allergic reactions, because the symptoms remain localized.

Allergic reactions are accompanied by symptoms that affect other areas of the body.

Mild allergic reactions are characterized by only a few noticeable signs of allergy, such as mildly flushed skin, a pronounced swelling (especially at the sting site), and hives. Although mild, this degree of reaction is an important warning signal and can occur up to 24 hours after the sting. The child's health care provider might prescribe an antihistamine to help control mild symptoms. Antihistamine in liquid form is easier for a young child to swallow, and it works more quickly inside the body than the pill form does.

Severe allergic reactions vary in intensity and usually occur within minutes after contact with the insect venom. The reaction can result in anaphylaxis and death if the necessary medication to reverse the reaction is not immediately available. See the section *Anaphylaxis* in Chapter 5.

Symptoms of a severe allergic reaction include:

- Hives with welts

- Dizziness

- Swelling at the sting site and face, tongue, and throat swelling

- Abdominal or stomach cramps and diarrhea

- Tightness in the chest

- Wheezing or difficulty breathing caused by swelling in the throat that can progress to a complete blockage of the airway

- Blue/gray color around lips and mouth

What to Do

1. Examine the sting site for a stinger. Only honey bees leave the stinger with the venom sac attached. It can continue to inject venom for 2 or 3 minutes if left in the skin. Scrape it away from the site with a fingernail, table knife blade, or similar object. Avoid using fingers or tweezers, because this squeezes the sac and injects more venom.

2. Apply a baking soda and water paste to reduce the stinging pain. Baking soda neutralizes acidic venom. If the insect was a wasp, put vinegar or lemon juice on the sting site to neutralize the alkaline venom. Later, apply calamine lotion to help control itching.

3. Apply ice or a cold pack wrapped in a wet cloth for 15 to 20 minutes to slow the absorption of venom and relieve pain.

4. Observe the child for signs of an allergic reaction. If a severe allergic reaction or anaphylaxis occurs:

   - Call EMS immediately for anaphylaxis.

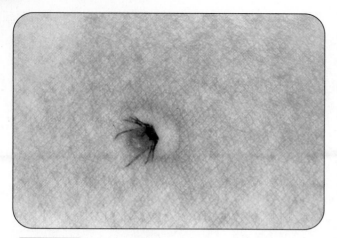

Figure 10-4) Embedded tick.

- Use a child's allergic emergency kit if you have it on hand and have been instructed in its use. At least one staff member in the center should be taught to use the kit. It should be stored with first aid supplies at room temperature. This is a prescription drug intended specifically for the allergic child. Older children should have their kit with them at all times. The kit contains an easy-to-use mechanism that administers the correct dose of the drug. A second dose of medication might be necessary.

- Check and monitor the ABCs and treat accordingly. Swelling in the throat makes rescue breathing difficult.

- Position an unresponsive but breathing child on his or her side (recovery position). Position a responsive child who is having difficulty breathing in a sitting position to make breathing easier.

- Position the sting site so that it is lower than the level of the heart.

Tick Bites

Most tick bites are harmless, although ticks occasionally carry diseases such as Rocky Mountain spotted fever and Lyme disease. Ticks attach themselves to clothing or the exposed skin of a person walking in the woods or tall grasses. A tick bite is often not felt and the tick can remain attached and embedded for days (▲ **Figure 10-4**).

Diseases are transmitted after the tick bites the skin and while it is feeding. As ticks draw blood for food, some can increase their size by 10 times (► **Figures 10-5 and 10-6**). Check children and pets regularly for ticks and remove them promptly (**Figure 10-7 ►**).

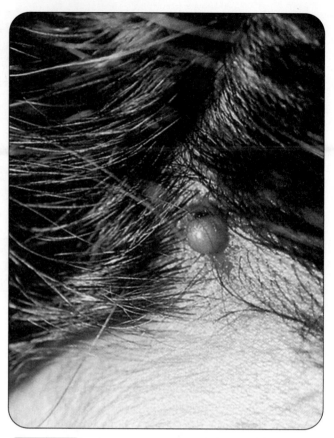

Figure 10-5) An engorged tick at the hair line.

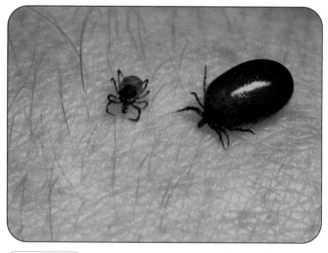

Figure 10-6) Unengorged and engorged deer ticks.

Removing Ticks

Use tweezers rather than fingertips to grasp the tick close to the skin surface. Do not attempt to remove a tick by coating it with petroleum jelly or fingernail polish or by holding a hot match against it. Pull gently and firmly until the tick lets go. Do not twist or jerk, because this might leave part of the tick in the skin. Wash the area with soap and water. Dab rubbing alcohol on the bite area. Apply calamine lotion for itching. Notify the child's parent at the end of the day.

Observe the bite site for a doughnut-shaped or other rash or signs of infection for the next several weeks. Also observe the child for flu-like symptoms such as fever, muscle aches, or joint pain and for sensitivity to bright light. The child's health care provider should be contacted about any symptoms that develop for up to 4 weeks after a tick bite (► Figure 10-8).

Tick Bite Prevention

- Cover legs with long pants tucked into socks, tuck in long-sleeved shirts at the waist, and wear sneakers instead of sandals when walking in tall grasses, woods, or fields. Ticks are most easily spotted on light-colored clothing.

- Stay on trails whenever possible.

- Check children's skin after playing in these areas. Pay special attention to the folds of the skin, the scalp, and the back of the neck. Removing the tick within the first 24 hours greatly reduces the risk of infection.

- Contact your local health department to find out if deer ticks are prevalent in your area.

- Check pets for ticks. They can carry ticks and are also susceptible to disease. Use tick control products recommended by your veterinarian.

- Parents may use over-the-counter insect repellents that contain no more than 10% DEET on infants and small children. DEET on the skin irritates ticks and causes them to drop off. A repellent containing 0.5% Permethrin, a pesticide, should be applied to the clothing only, never to the skin. Child care providers should not expose children in their care to situations where the use of DEET would be necessary.

- Spray insect repellents only when outdoors, use sparingly, and wash hands after applying. Never apply them to the face, to an open wound or cut, or to the hands or arms of a child who is likely to put them in the mouth.

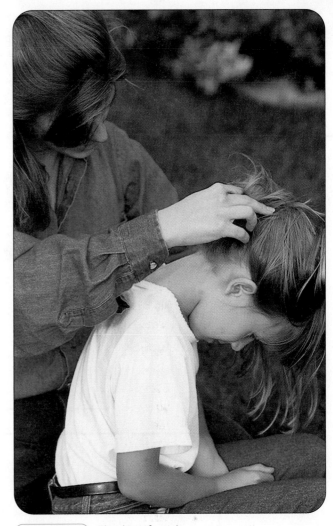

Figure 10-7 Checking for ticks.

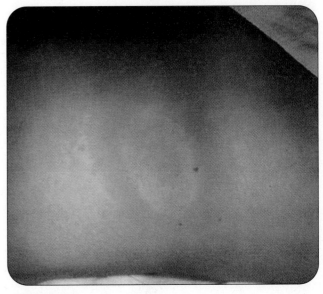

Figure 10-8 Lyme disease rash.

INSECT STINGS

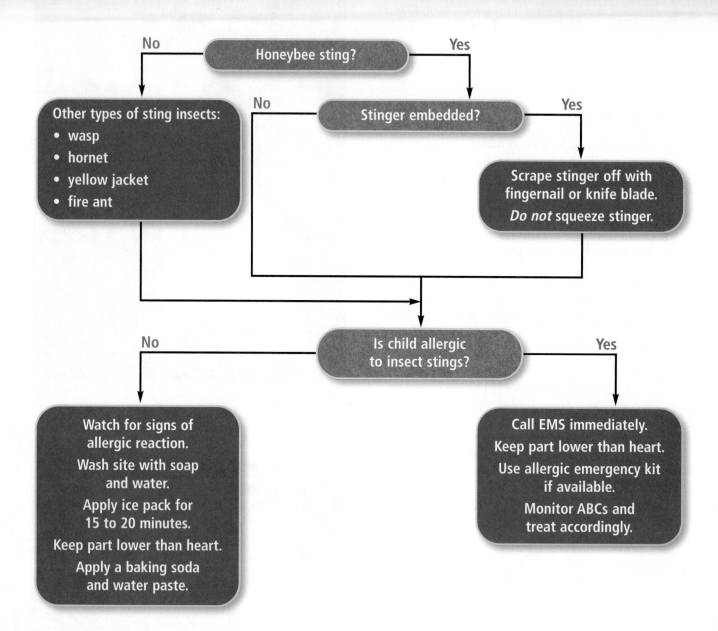

Honeybee sting?

No → **Other types of sting insects:**
- wasp
- hornet
- yellow jacket
- fire ant

Yes → **Stinger embedded?**

No

Yes → **Scrape stinger off with fingernail or knife blade. *Do not* squeeze stinger.**

Is child allergic to insect stings?

No → **Watch for signs of allergic reaction.**

Wash site with soap and water.

Apply ice pack for 15 to 20 minutes.

Keep part lower than heart.

Apply a baking soda and water paste.

Yes → **Call EMS immediately.**

Keep part lower than heart.

Use allergic emergency kit if available.

Monitor ABCs and treat accordingly.

Avoiding Insect Stings

There are ways for children and staff to reduce the chance of being stung while outdoors. These are especially important for the allergic child.

+ Destroy any nests around the building. Check under eaves and windowsills.

+ Check for nests in other locations where children play such as in old tree stumps, in auto tires that are part of a playground, in holes in the ground, and around rotting wood.

+ Allergic children should not play outside alone when stinging insects are active.

+ Sneakers are safer than sandals in preventing foot stings.

+ Clothing for allergic children should not have bright floral prints; white or khaki is best. Avoid loose-fitting clothes.

+ Avoid perfumes, hairsprays, or other products with scents.

+ When eating outdoors, know that these foods especially attract insects: tuna, peanut butter and jelly sandwiches, watermelon, sweetened beverages, and ice cream.

+ Avoid garbage cans and dumpsters.

+ If an insect is near you, do not swat or run; such actions can trigger an attack. Walk away slowly. If you have disturbed a nest and the insects swarm around you, lie face down and cover your head with your arms. Teach this technique to children.

+ An allergic child should wear a medical alert necklace or bracelet.

Did You Know?

Allergy to *Hymenoptera* insect venom is not an inherited trait. A child does not have an increased risk for developing this allergy if a parent or sibling is allergic.

The Soft Drink Can Sting

Children who are playing outdoors and walk away from their soft drink or juice cans might receive an unpleasant surprise when they come back for another sip. A stinging insect, attracted to the sweetness of the soda, can end up in the child's mouth. A sting in this location can cause the throat to swell even in a nonallergic child.

As an ounce of prevention, pour beverages into clear plastic cups when outdoors. This way, the child can see that no insects are in the beverage.

Should a sting occur inside the mouth, give the child plenty of ice chips to suck on for pain relief. Avoid using ice cubes with young children because they are slippery and can block the airway. If you know it is a bee sting, have the child repeatedly rinse the mouth with a mixture of 1 teaspoon of baking soda in 8 ounces of water to help neutralize the acid venom.

Keep Kids and Snakes Apart

Poisonous snakes exist in all parts of the United States but are a problem only in areas with large numbers of them.

+ Be aware of the poisonous species in your area, and avoid taking young children to locations near woods, grasses, or desert where snakes live.

+ Teach children not to poke into crevices or holes, under rocks, or around logs.

+ Do not allow children to tease or poke at a snake, even a dead one.

+ If you come upon a snake you believe to be poisonous, immediately retrace your steps in the opposite direction or make a very large circle around it.

+ Let a snake know you are coming by making noise as you walk along.

Learning Activities

Bites and Stings

Directions: Circle Yes if you agree with the statement, and circle No if you disagree.

Yes No **1.** An animal bite that does not break the skin can become infected.

Yes No **2.** Both warm-blooded and cold-blooded animals can become infected with rabies.

Yes No **3.** Family pets are the leading rabies carriers.

Yes No **4.** The rabies virus is passed through the saliva of an infected animal.

Yes No **5.** A small amount of bleeding while washing a bite wound helps to clean it.

Yes No **6.** Unneutered dogs are more likely to bite than neutered dogs.

Yes No **7.** Place a warm pack over a sting site to decrease the pain.

Yes No **8.** The yellow jacket is the only insect that leaves a stinger in the skin.

Yes No **9.** A baking soda and water paste helps to relieve the pain of a sting by neutralizing acidic venom.

Yes No **10.** The likelihood of infection from a human bite is greater than from an animal bite.

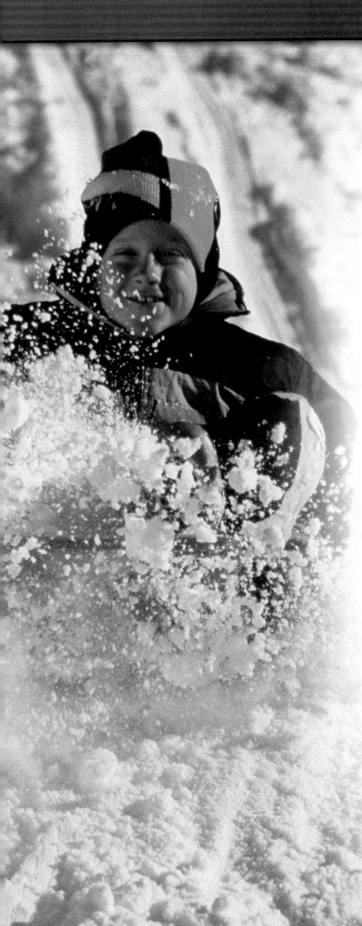

Chapter 11

Heat and Cold Emergencies

Cold-Related Emergencies

Children should be encouraged to play outdoors even during the colder weather months. However, some winter weather conditions can sneak up on a lost child or a child busily intent on play and have dangerous consequences to health.

Frostbite and Frostnip

Frostbite occurs when skin and underlying tissues are damaged by exposure to below-freezing temperatures. As the tissue freezes, the blood circulation slows, reducing the amount of oxygen that gets to the tissues. Both air temperature and length of exposure determine the extent of the damage.

Frostbite is often seen on hands, cheeks, ears, noses, and feet. Children are more susceptible to frostbite than adults, because they have less body fat to insulate them.

Frostnip occurs on the same areas as frostbite, but is less serious than frostbite because the damage does not penetrate as deeply. If ignored, frostnip can develop into frostbite.

What to Look For

Initially, the affected area feels cold and mildly painful to the child who is outdoors and focused on play or other activity. The pain subsides as the skin becomes numb, if exposure continues. The following signs and symptoms are most apparent when the child comes indoors:

- Coldness and numbness

- Tingling and burning

- Aching or throbbing pain

- Milky-white or grayish-yellow skin color

Dressing for Winter

+ Mittens keep hands warmer than gloves.

+ Wear insulated and water-repellent boots and snowpants.

+ Wear a hat because a large percentage of body heat loss occurs through the head.

+ Apply petroleum jelly to exposed areas of the face to prevent chapping.

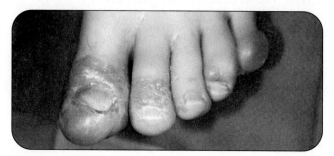

Figure 11-1 Blistered, frostbitten toes.

As exposure to the cold increases, these signs of more severe frostbite appear:

- Skin blisters ▲ **Figure 11-1**
- Swelling of affected area
- Skin that feels hard

What to Do

1. Bring the child indoors and remove clothing and jewelry from the affected area.

2. Handle the area very gently while you examine it.

3. Allow the area to warm on its own. If symptoms persist or signs of more serious frostbite develop, have the child seen in an emergency medical facility.

Caution:

DO NOT rub snow on the affected area.

DO NOT rub the area to stimulate circulation. This could further damage fragile skin.

DO NOT break blisters on frostbitten skin.

DO NOT allow a child to walk if his or her feet might be frostbitten.

DO NOT attempt to warm the affected area by using warm water, a heating pad, or a blow dryer.

Preventing Frostbite and Frostnip

Frostbite and frostnip occur when children are playing outdoors or enjoying winter sports for long periods of time, are inadequately dressed for the cold, and fail to notice their developing symptoms. Take the following precautions to prevent either of these conditions from occurring:

+ Dress appropriately. See the section *Dressing for Winter* in this chapter.

+ Observe for white spots forming on cheeks that might indicate mild frostbite.

+ Bring a child indoors immediately if he or she complains of a cold, numb, tingling, or painful area on the body.

+ Check the temperature and limit outdoor play time accordingly during the cold-weather months.

+ Teach children about the importance of frostbite prevention—once frostbitten, the injured part is more susceptible to future episodes of frostbite and continues to be extremely sensitive to cold. The child can experience tingling, loss of feeling, and pain during cold weather for many years.

Hypothermia

Hypothermia is a dangerous condition in which the body loses more heat than it can produce, causing the core body temperature to drop below 95°F. It is caused by prolonged exposure to cold air or cold water. Hypothermia slows the activity of all body tissues and can be life-threatening. Children are especially susceptible to hypothermia because they have less fat than adults.

A child who becomes hypothermic is outdoors for a very long time and/or is inadequately prepared for the weather conditions. If a child falls through ice or is separated from adults on a walk and spends several hours outdoors before being rescued, hypothermia may be accompanied by frostbite.

Even during summer, hypothermia is a danger. Swimmers who stay in the water too long and children wearing light clothing who are caught in wet and windy weather are especially susceptible. Wet conditions, whether from rain, snow, or perspiration, increase heat loss from the body and are often associated with hypothermia. A 50°F temperature in wet conditions is more dangerous than a 20°F temperature in dry conditions. Wind also increases heat loss, so pay attention to the wind-chill factor when making outdoor plans in winter.

FROSTBITE

Remove child
from cold exposure
if possible.

Remove clothing or
jewelry from
affected part(s).

Do not rub.
Put dry, clean gauze
or cloth between
fingers and toes, and
over broken blisters.

Seek medical
attention.

HYPOTHERMIA

Move child into
a warm area.

Handle child
gently.

Replace wet clothing
with dry clothing
or coverings.

Insulate child
from cold.

Seek immediate
medical attention.

Heat stroke
- Dry, flushed, hot skin
- Very high body temperature
- No sweating
- Life-threatening

Heat exhaustion
- Moist, pale, cool skin
- Normal or sub-normal temperature
- Heavy sweating
- Serious, but not life-threatening

105°F+ ——   —— 98.6°F

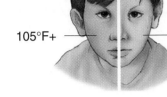

Figure 11-2 Comparison of heat stroke and heat exhaustion.

Heat-Related Emergencies

Most children love the summer and the seemingly endless hours of outdoor play. Being outdoors provides many health benefits, yet it is important to know that the sun and the heat can be dangerous. Use common sense and follow the recommendations in this section to avoid heat-related injuries, caused by overexposure to high temperatures. These injuries can be mild or life-threatening, depending on the degree of heat and the length of time that the child is exposed (▲ **Figure 11-2**).

Heat Stroke

Heat stroke is the most severe heat illness and is a life-threatening emergency. It occurs when a person is exposed to or exerts himself in a very high environmental temperature. When this happens, the body's heat-regulating ability becomes overwhelmed and ceases to function properly, resulting in an inability to sweat and a dangerously high rise in body temperature. Heat stroke can

develop suddenly. Brain, liver, and kidney damage and death can result if the body is not cooled immediately. Hospitalization is always necessary.

What to Look For

- Body temperature approaching 106°F or higher
- Very hot and dry skin
- Skin flushed (bright red face in light-skinned children)
- Rapid breathing and pulse
- Confusion, delirium
- Loss of consciousness

What to Do

Begin first aid immediately. The longer it takes to start treatment, the more likely it is that there will be serious complications or death.

1. Call EMS.
2. Move the child to a cool place.
3. Check and monitor the ABCs and treat as needed.
4. Remove outer clothing, such as shirt and pants.
5. Begin cooling the child while waiting for EMS to arrive. Place ice packs wrapped in a cloth on body areas with abundant blood supply such as the armpits, groin, and neck. Also spray or pour cold water over the child. Fan the child to speed the evaporation of water, which is effective in reducing temperature.
6. Have the child seen in an emergency medical facility immediately.

In the News

Exposure to cold slows activity in the body's tissues and decreases their demand for oxygen. Normally, the heart and brain cannot survive undamaged for more than a few minutes without oxygen. But in a hypothermic state, they need so little oxygen that, under certain conditions, they can remain undamaged for up to an hour. This may explain why some children have survived near-drowning accidents in very cold water. However, although well-publicized, these incidents happen infrequently.

The Short Errand Mistake

A pleasant, sunny day of 78°F with a gentle breeze is hardly the day that we think about heat stroke. However, even at this comfortable temperature, the air temperature inside a closed car parked in the sun can reach 120°F in less than 20 minutes. Do not leave a child in a closed car while you run into a store, even for just a few minutes. If you see a child left unattended in a closed car, alert the local police. If the car is unlocked, open the door and check on the child.

HEAT-RELATED EMERGENCIES

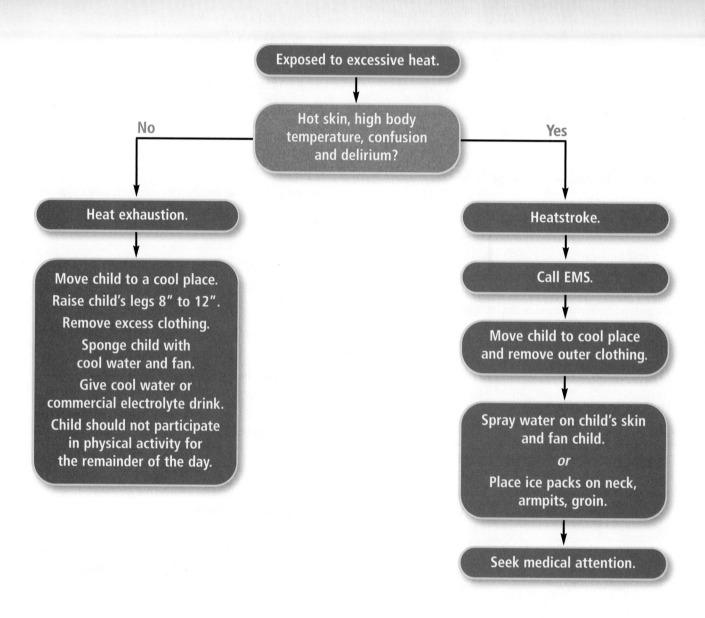

Exposed to excessive heat.

Hot skin, high body temperature, confusion and delirium?

No

Heat exhaustion.

Move child to a cool place.

Raise child's legs 8" to 12".

Remove excess clothing.

Sponge child with cool water and fan.

Give cool water or commercial electrolyte drink.

Child should not participate in physical activity for the remainder of the day.

Yes

Heatstroke.

Call EMS.

Move child to cool place and remove outer clothing.

Spray water on child's skin and fan child.

or

Place ice packs on neck, armpits, groin.

Seek medical attention.

Caution:

DO NOT place a semiconscious or unconscious child in the bathtub or give the child anything to eat or drink.

DO NOT give aspirin, acetaminophen, or ibuprofen in an attempt to reduce the temperature. These medications will have no effect.

Preventing Heat-Related Emergencies

(Also see *Sunburn Precautions* in Chapter 6).

+ Encourage children to drink cool water frequently. Fruit juices and popsicles are fine hot weather treats. Also encourage salty snacks such as pretzels and crackers. Do not give salt tablets. Salt is best consumed mixed with water as a drink.

+ Avoid vigorous physical activity during the midday hours when temperatures are usually the highest.

+ Provide cooling activities such as a sprinkler or a wading pool on hot days.

+ Dress children in lightweight and loose-fitting clothing in hot weather.

+ Never leave a child in a closed vehicle in warm weather.

Heat Exhaustion

Heat exhaustion occurs when the body loses too much water and salt through sweating. In children, it is often the result of prolonged physical activity in high temperatures without pauses for drinking enough water. This condition differs from heat stroke in that the child sweats heavily, the body temperature remains normal, and the child's mental status remains clear. Heat exhaustion is less critical than heat stroke, but it requires prompt attention.

What to Look For

- Normal body temperature
- Skin pale and clammy, with heavy sweating
- Fast and weak pulse
- Tiredness and weakness
- Headache, dizziness, and feeling faint
- Thirst
- Nausea and vomiting
- Muscle cramps
- Alert and aware

What to Do

1. Move the child to a cool place to rest.
2. Have the child drink a glass of cool water (lightly salted) or a commercial sports drink. If you do not have salt available, cold tap water alone is helpful.
3. Raise the child's legs 8″ to 12″.
4. Sponge the child with cool, wet cloths on the head, face, and trunk, and fan the child.
5. The child must not participate in physical activity for the rest of the day.

Heat Cramps

Heat cramps are painful spasms in muscles that cause a temporary loss of mobility. They are caused by the loss of water and possibly also by the loss of salt through heavy sweating. This results in inadequate circulation of blood to the major leg and abdominal muscles used in exercise or play. The cramping can last from a few minutes to several hours. Heat cramps are never serious by themselves but can be one of the symptoms of heat exhaustion, a more serious heat-related illness.

What to Look For

- Painful cramping of the muscle
- Heavy sweating
- Thirst

What to Do

1. Get the child into a comfortable position.
2. Give the child a glass of cool water (lightly salted) or a commercial sports drink, half-strength and diluted with water. Do not give more than three glasses and give them at 15-minute intervals.
3. Gently stretch the muscle.

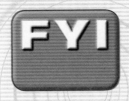 Drinking one to two glasses of water during the hour before vigorous outdoor play or sports and taking water breaks while exercising can help prevent heat cramps.

Learning Activities

Heat and Cold Emergencies

Directions: Circle Yes if you agree with the statement, and circle No if you disagree.

Yes No **1.** Frostbite is seen most often on the hands, nose, and feet.

Yes No **2.** Massage the frostbitten area to help restore circulation.

Yes No **3.** Wrap frostbitten fingers snuggly together to speed rewarming.

Yes No **4.** Once frostbitten, a body part is more susceptible to future episodes of frostbite.

Yes No **5.** Hypothermia occurs only in the winter.

Yes No **6.** Gloves keep fingers warmer than mittens.

Yes No **7.** Shivering increases the body temperature.

Yes No **8.** Heat stroke is a life-threatening emergency.

Yes No **9.** Aspirin or acetaminophen is helpful in treating heat stroke, but not heat exhaustion.

Yes No **10.** Heat cramps are caused by a loss of water and salt through heavy sweating.

Yes No **11.** The most effective way to cool a child with heat stroke is to use cool water and fanning.

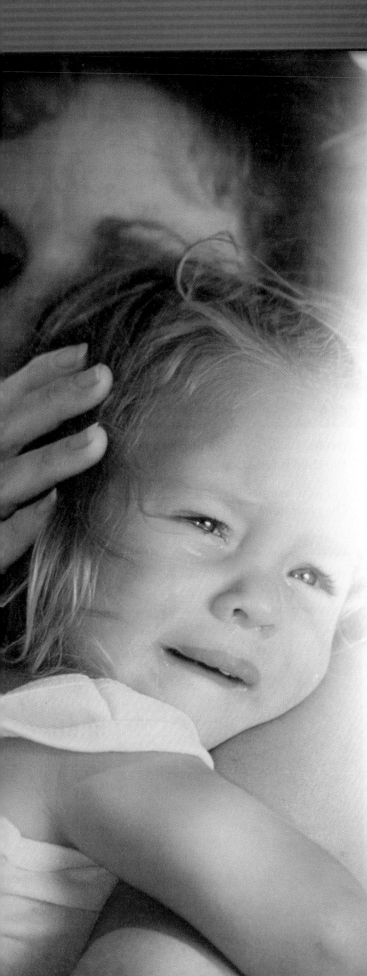

Chapter 12

Sudden Illnesses

Croup

Croup—an acute swelling of the vocal cords caused by a viral infection—is common in infants and young children. It is not a disease, but a group of respiratory symptoms that lasts for 3 to 5 days, and can usually be treated at home.

An attack of croup typically occurs suddenly; the child may awaken from sleep with a hoarse, barking cough and difficulty breathing. The child has flaring nostrils and works very hard to breathe, sometimes using the neck and abdominal muscles. Often the nose and lips have a blue or gray discoloration. Usually there is no fever.

What to Do

Hold the child on your lap, along with a favorite book or stuffed animal, in front of a cool mist vaporizer and have the child breathe in the mist. This misting helps to decrease the swelling in the air passages. Taking the child into the bathroom and turning on the shower produces the same effect. The child's breathing should show signs of improvement in 10 to 15 minutes. If the child continues to have difficulty breathing after this treatment, call the child's parent or health care provider.

Dehydration

Dehydration is an excessive loss of fluids from the body. It occurs when the total amount of water lost through sweating, urination, diarrhea, and vomiting is greater than the fluids taken in. Fever, vomiting, diarrhea, and heat exhaustion are especially worrisome in infants and young children because they can lead to dehydration. A child with severe dehydration must be hospitalized to receive intravenous fluids.

When a child is sick, offer frequent sips of clear fluids. See clear fluid suggestions in *Vomiting*, in Chapter 16. Even the most diligent child care provider sometimes has difficulty getting a child to drink if the child has a sore throat.

What to Look For

- A decreased amount of urine that has a dark color and a strong odor, because it is concentrated
- No tears when crying
- Dry, cracked lips with little or no saliva
- Sunken eyes
- Listlessness, sleepiness
- Poor skin turgor—to determine this, lightly pull up a fold of skin and release it. Skin with poor turgor returns slowly to normal position or remains "tented."
- A sunken fontanel (soft spot) in an infant under 1 year of age

What to Do

Call the parent if the child shows any signs of dehydration. A parent should contact the health care provider if the child:

- has been unable to drink for several hours as a result of illness, especially if the child is an infant under 6 months of age.
- has had several episodes of vomiting and diarrhea.
- has had watery diarrhea for 2 to 3 days.

Fainting

Fainting is a sudden and temporary loss of consciousness caused by a brief lack of blood and oxygen to the brain. Fainting is not caused by an injury; it is a nervous system reaction to such situations as fear, pain, or a strong emotional upset. Occasionally, prolonged standing in a warm environment results in fainting.

What to Look For

Signs and symptoms that a child is about to faint include:

- Lightheadedness and dizziness
- Nausea
- Pale skin color
- Sweating

What to Do

1. Lay the child on the back to prevent falling. If the child has already fainted, position the child on the back (▶ **Figure 12-1**).
2. Elevate the legs 8″ to 12″ to increase blood flow to the brain.
3. Loosen tight-fitting clothing.
4. Apply a cool, wet cloth to the face.
5. Check for injuries that might have occurred if the child fell.

A child who has fainted recovers quickly, often in 1 to 2 minutes. Fainting is generally not serious and, in children, can usually be traced to a triggering event. You should call EMS if the child remains unconscious. A health care provider should see a child who has repeated attacks of fainting for no apparent reason.

Some young children cause themselves to faint by holding their breath. These breath-holding spells are often caused by frustration, anger, and sometimes fear. Uncontrolled crying is followed by breath holding until the child loses consciousness. The child begins to breathe spontaneously after fainting and regains consciousness within several seconds. There is no specific treatment, and the episodes disappear as the child matures. A parent might want to discuss the problem with the child's health care provider.

Caution:

DO NOT give anything to eat or drink until the child is fully alert.

DO NOT use smelling salts or ammonia. They irritate the lining of the airway.

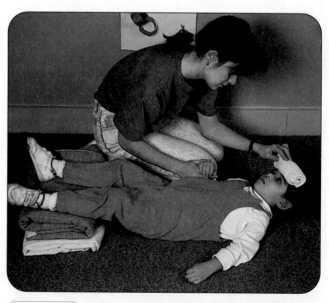

(**Figure 12-1**) Positioning of a child who has fainted.

Near-Drowning

Drowning is a leading cause of injury resulting in death among children. More than one half of all drownings happen to children 5 years of age and under. Drowning can be a silent killer, and it can happen quickly. Equally sad are the near-drowning victims who survive but suffer brain damage and a reduced quality of life. Near-drowning refers to surviving a prolonged period of time under water without oxygen.

A drowning or a near-drowning can occur in any body of water in which the nose and mouth of a child can be submerged. Obviously, it's important to be cautious in and around large bodies of deep water. But remember that drownings can also occur in toilets, bathtubs, sinks, water buckets, fish tanks, and wading pools with only inches of water.

What to Do

1. Send someone to call for EMS.

2. Rescue the child from the water. If you suspect that a spinal injury has occurred because the child is unconscious or is injured after a dive, keep the head, neck, and spine straight. To do this, float the child onto a large full-body board and lift the child out of the water gently, supporting the head and neck.

3. Establish consciousness, check the ABCs and treat, as needed. If you are alone and must perform either rescue breathing or CPR, do so for 1 minute before stopping to call EMS yourself.

4. If the child vomits, which is likely after a near-drowning, roll the child onto the left side as 1 unit to avoid twisting the neck and spine. This position allows vomit to drain and keeps the airway open.

Although infrequent, successful rescues have occurred after prolonged submersions in cold water. This is because the body's oxygen requirement is reduced in cold water, making it possible for the brain to survive longer without oxygen than the standard 4 to 6 minutes. See *Water Safety,* Chapter 17.

Seizures

A seizure, or convulsion, is a disturbance in the electrical impulses of the brain. Such disturbances result in a variety of body responses. These range from the very mild, such as a few moments of staring, to the more severe collapse with loss of consciousness, and the strong shaking of large voluntary muscles. Causes of seizures, other than a seizure disorder, include: high fever, head injury, serious illness, and poisoning. A person who experiences a seizure for the first time should always receive immediate emergency medical care.

Sometimes a specific cause of the seizure can be identified, but more commonly, the cause remains unknown. Even without knowing the exact cause, a health care provider can usually treat the child with medication to control the seizures or reduce their frequency.

The most easily recognizable seizure, and one for which first aid care is helpful, involves the entire body, and is called a *grand mal* seizure. When a seizure is about to happen, an older, experienced child might be able to recognize specific symptoms, known as an "aura." This is an internal warning system, which can be a noise, visual change, funny taste, numbness, or other feeling, that causes the child to know that a seizure is about to occur. Some children experience no aura, or cannot recognize it as such, and do not know that the seizure is about to start.

What to Look For

• Loss of consciousness

• Breathing that stops temporarily

• Rigid body with jerking and shaking movements

• Neck and back arching

• Eyes rolling back

• Increased saliva production causing drooling or foaming at the mouth

• Incontinence of urine or stool

The uncontrolled movements of a child having a seizure can be frightening to watch. A seizure must run its course. There is nothing you can do to interrupt it or stop it.

What to Do

1. Position the child on the side (recovery position) to allow saliva to drain and to keep the tongue from blocking the airway.

2. Move toys and furniture out of the way.

3. Slide the palm of your hand under the child's head to protect it.

4. Time the seizure and observe the body parts affected. A seizure might seem to last longer than it actually does, especially if you are frightened. Your detailed description is important to the child's health care provider.

5. Call EMS if child has no seizure history.

SEIZURES

Seizure.

Turn child onto left side.

Move away toys
and furniture.

Protect child's head
with your hand.

Time and observe
the seizure.

Look for medical-alert
identification tag
(bracelet or necklace).

Do not give child
anything to drink or eat.

Do not put anything between
child's teeth.

Seek medical attention if
child has no history of seizures.

Otherwise, follow child's
seizure care plan.

6. Let the child rest in the recovery position after the seizure. Recovery from a seizure is slow and the child will sleep or be drowsy for a while.

7. Check for a medical alert tag that might identify a seizure disorder.

8. A child who is known to have seizures should have a treatment plan. Follow this plan and call the child's parent.

Caution:

DO NOT force anything between the child's teeth.

DO NOT restrain the child's movements.

DO NOT give anything to eat or drink until the child is fully alert.

Febrile Seizures

In a small percentage of children, a rapid rise in fever can cause a *grand mal* seizure. A febrile seizure is not related to a chronic seizure disorder and has no effect on the child's neurologic development or brain function.

A febrile seizure rarely occurs in children under 6 months of age and is most common between 18 months and 3 years of age. It seldom occurs in children over 6 years of age. A child who has experienced a febrile seizure is more likely to have another one.

Treat a febrile seizure as you would any *grand mal* seizure. A child who has a febrile seizure for the first time should be seen in an emergency medical facility immediately. If the child has experienced a febrile seizure, the parent should speak with the child's health care provider about what can be done to reduce the likelihood of another seizure.

Sudden Infant Death Syndrome (SIDS) and Infant Apnea*

Sudden Infant Death Syndrome (SIDS) is the sudden and unexpected death of an apparently healthy infant, which cannot be explained by autopsy or by the child's health history. It is a leading cause of death in babies under 1 year of age, with most infant victims being between 2 and 4 months of age. SIDS crosses all racial and socioeconomic boundaries. Most SIDS deaths occur during the night or at nap time, and the greatest number of cases occur in the winter months. Often the infant had a viral respiratory illness 1 to 2 weeks before the death.

The exact causes of SIDS are not yet understood. SIDS researchers are working to discover a means of early detection and prevention as well as the underlying causes. This involves learning more about how a healthy infant develops and functions. No association has ever been found between SIDS and childhood immunizations.

Because studies showed that young infants put to bed on the stomach had a greater incidence of SIDS than those who were put to bed on the side or back, it is now strongly recommended that infants always be put to sleep on the back in all settings, including the crib, stroller, and playpen. In 1992, the nationwide Back to Sleep recommendation was initiated, and, since then, the incidence of SIDS has decreased by 43%. Parents and child care providers need to know that the back sleeping position offers the lowest risk of SIDS.

It is also recommended that:

+ young infants sleep on a firm mattress in a standard size crib.

+ no pillows, comforters, stuffed animals, or any other soft bedding be in the crib.

+ young infants never be put to sleep on a water bed.

When a baby dies of SIDS, parents or child care providers often blame themselves, but it is no one's fault. It could not have been prevented. In fact, in the few observed cases of deaths attributed to SIDS, CPR techniques were unsuccessful in resuscitating the infants. Support groups are available for families who have suffered the loss of an infant to SIDS. Health care providers can help parents find a SIDS support group.

Another condition of infancy that can be confused with SIDS is infant apnea. Apnea is a temporary stoppage of breathing. Only a tiny percentage of SIDS victims experience episodes of apnea before death.

Short periods of apnea—less than 15 seconds—are normal and safe. Many infants pause in their breathing in this manner. Apnea becomes life threatening when it is prolonged. Prolonged apnea can cause the infant to choke or gag and to become limp. The skin color can become pale and blue or gray. Many children with prolonged infant apnea respond successfully to CPR. Most infants outgrow apnea by 6 months of age.

Adapted from "Facts on Sudden Infant Death Syndrome," courtesy of the Sudden Infant Death Syndrome Alliance.

Learning Activities

Sudden Illnesses

Directions: Circle Yes if you agree with the statement, and circle No if you disagree.

Yes No **1.** A child with dehydration has dark, concentrated urine.

Yes No **2.** A child who has fainted should regain consciousness within 5 to 10 minutes.

Yes No **3.** A seizure can be caused by a rapid rise in fever, a head injury, serious illness, or poisoning.

Yes No **4.** First aid for a seizure includes placing a firm object between the teeth.

Yes No **5.** A victim of infant apnea will not respond to CPR.

Yes No **6.** Place a child having a seizure in the shock position.

Yes No **7.** Use a cool mist vaporizer or shower mist to help a child with croup breathe more easily.

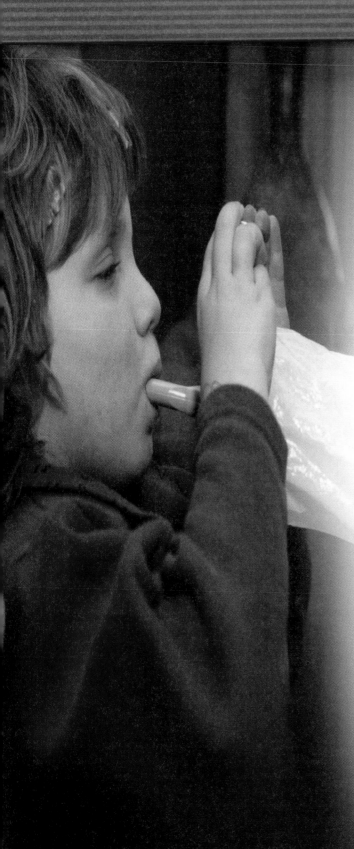

Chapter 13

Children with Medical Conditions that Affect Child Care

Asthma

Asthma is a common chronic disease of childhood, affecting more than 5 million children. According to the American Lung Association, asthma is on the increase in both children and adults, as a result of increased exposure to environmental pollutants and irritants. The American Academy of Allergy, Asthma, and Immunology estimates that annually, children with asthma make more than 2.7 million visits to their health care providers and require 200,000 hospitalizations. Asthma also accounts for 10 million school absences each year.

The sporadic breathing difficulties that a child with asthma experiences are often called "attacks". During these attacks, the lining of the airways throughout the lungs swells and narrows. The normal production of mucus increases, further narrowing the airway. Additionally, the muscles surrounding the chest tighten, making breathing difficult. Some children experience an annoying chronic cough; others experience sudden attacks with breathing difficulty so severe that they cannot complete a sentence.

In some children, asthma is so mild that it is termed hidden, and the disease can go unnoticed. Commonly, these children have frequent upper respiratory infections and mild coughs. Their inability to take long, deep breaths often prohibits them from participating in vigorous activity.

Asthma Triggers

Children with asthma develop respiratory symptoms when they are exposed to various allergens and irritants. These substances are called asthma triggers (Figure 13-1 ▶).

Children must be taught which allergic substances and irritants trigger their asthma attacks and how to avoid them so that they can start sharing the responsibility for monitoring and managing their health condition.

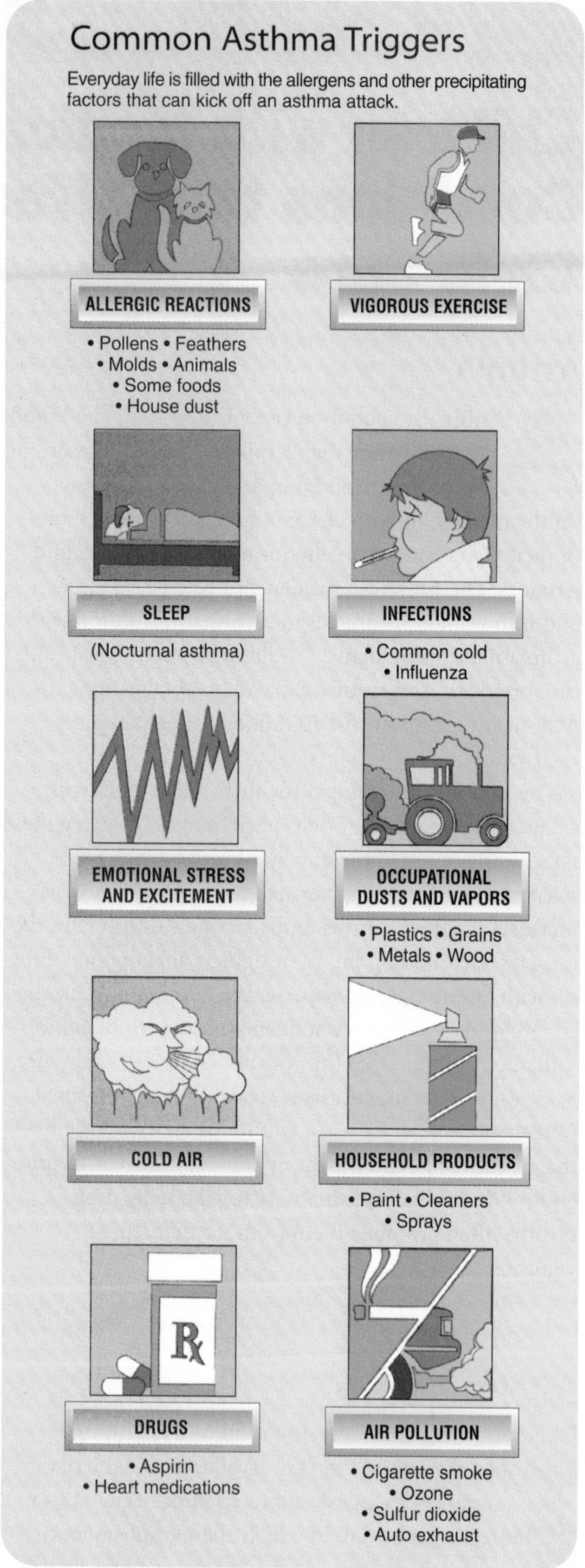

Common Asthma Triggers

Everyday life is filled with the allergens and other precipitating factors that can kick off an asthma attack.

ALLERGIC REACTIONS
• Pollens • Feathers
• Molds • Animals
• Some foods
• House dust

VIGOROUS EXERCISE

SLEEP
(Nocturnal asthma)

INFECTIONS
• Common cold
• Influenza

EMOTIONAL STRESS AND EXCITEMENT

OCCUPATIONAL DUSTS AND VAPORS
• Plastics • Grains
• Metals • Wood

COLD AIR

HOUSEHOLD PRODUCTS
• Paint • Cleaners
• Sprays

DRUGS
• Aspirin
• Heart medications

AIR POLLUTION
• Cigarette smoke
• Ozone
• Sulfur dioxide
• Auto exhaust

Figure 13-1 Source: American Lung Association®— The "Christmas Seal People.®"

Asthma Care Plan

Managing a child's asthma is a daily consideration. Asthma conditions vary widely among children, making it imperative that each child have an individualized asthma care plan supplied by the child's parent or health care provider. Each child with asthma has unique needs and a child care provider must be able to respond to those needs. This plan should include:

1. A description of the child's asthma triggers and activities that the child should avoid.
2. A list of the child's medications with an explanation of why they are given.
3. A written explanation describing symptoms of the child's asthma attack and how to treat them.
4. A typical peak flow meter level if the child uses a peak flow meter. A peak flow meter is a simple device that measures the volume of air that can be expelled from the lungs in one breath.
5. Emergency telephone numbers if the parent is unavailable.

Symptoms of a Developing Asthma Attack

- Coughing. Coughing is the body's response to an irritation in the airway. A child with asthma eventually learns how to cough up mucus to clear the airway. Coughing increases when the child lays down.
- Wheezing. Wheezing is caused by narrowing of the airway and is heard on inhalation and exhalation.
- Chest tightness and shortness of breath. This is especially common following vigorous exercise. During a severe attack, the child's nostrils flare, and abdominal and neck muscles are used to help pull air into the lungs.
- Increased pulse and respiratory rate
- Pale skin color
- Fatigue
- Restlessness

What to Do

1. Take the child to a comfortable area where you can sit quietly.
2. Remove irritants or asthma triggers that might be affecting the child, such as an animal, smoke, or a strong perfume smell.
3. Give the child's asthma medication as prescribed by the child's health care provider. See *Using an Inhaler* in this chapter.

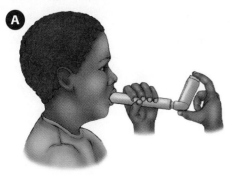
Using an inhaler and a holding chamber.

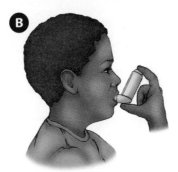
Using an inhaler by placing it in the mouth.

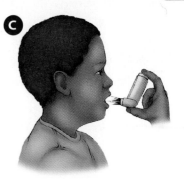
Using an inhaler by misting it 1–2 inches in front of the mouth.

Figure 13-2 A-C There are several methods for using air inhalers depending upon the age of the child and the type of medication. The method should be part of a child's asthma care plan.

4. Encourage the child to drink plenty of clear fluids to help thin the mucus in the lungs and make it easier for the child to cough up the secretions.

5. Keep the child at rest until he or she is breathing comfortably and feeling better.

6. Thoroughly document the event and the care you provide. See the *Documenting an Illness* form in Chapter 2.

7. Call the child's parent to notify the health care provider if the child's breathing does not improve within 5 to 10 minutes after you have administered the child's medication. You might be requested to administer another dose of medicine.

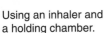
Caution:

DO NOT give asthma medications more often than prescribed.

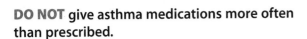

Call EMS if, after receiving medication:

- the child's breathing becomes more difficult.
- the child's lips or fingernails are blue/gray.
- the child is struggling to breathe, with flaring nostrils and strained muscles in the neck and abdomen.
- the child is unable to speak.
- the child appears exhausted.

Notify the child's parent that emergency medical help has been called.

Using an Inhaler

1. Hold the inhaler upright and shake it.

2. Remove the cap and place the inhaler into the holding chamber. The holding chamber is recommended for young children because it makes breathing the medicine easier. Other ways of delivering the medicine through an inhaler include placing the inhaler directly into the child's mouth or spraying the medication 1″ to 2″ in front of the child's mouth immediately prior to inhalation. The child's parent should leave instructions on how to use the inhaler (▲ **Figures 13-2 A-C**).

3. Have the child stand and tilt the head backward slightly because it is easiest to take a deep breath in this position. Instruct the child to empty the lungs by breathing out through the mouth.

4. Press down on the inhaler to release the medication at the same time as the child begins to inhale. Press down on the inhaler only once per breath.

5. Have the child breathe in through the mouth slowly and deeply and hold the breath for 10 seconds. This allows the medication to reach deep within the lungs.

6. Wait for at least 1 minute before administering a second puff of the medicine, if a second dose is prescribed.

Common side effects of asthma medicines include nervousness, shakiness, and a feeling that the heart is beating rapidly (see *Managing Asthma with Medications* in this chapter). These side effects should pass within 15 to 20 minutes. Never give more medicine than is prescribed by the child's health care provider because this could increase the side effects.

ASTHMA

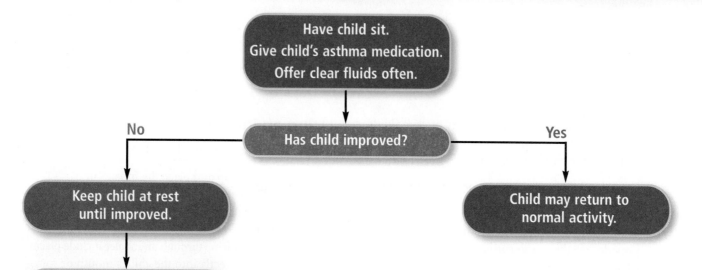

Have child sit.
Give child's asthma medication.
Offer clear fluids often.

Has child improved?

No

Yes

Keep child at rest until improved.

Child may return to normal activity.

Call for emergency medical help if, after receiving medication:

- the child's breathing becomes more difficult.
- the child's lips or fingernails are blue/gray.
- the child is struggling to breathe.
- the child is unable to speak.
- the child appears exhausted.

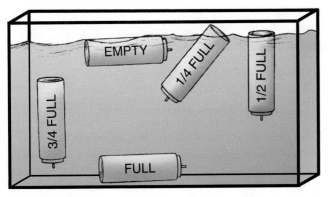

Figure 13-3 To determine how much medicine is in the inhaler, place it in a container of water and watch how it floats.

Cleaning and Care of an Inhaler

1. Clean the plastic mouth piece of the inhaler and the spacer or holding chamber with mild soap and warm water daily; let them air dry.

2. Keep an inhaler out of the reach of children, as you would any medication.

3. Alert the child's parents when the inhaler is ¼ full so a refill can be obtained (▲ **Figure 13-3**).

Using a Nebulizer

1. Choose a quiet and comfortable place for the child to sit. Wash your hands.

2. Measure the prescribed amount of medicine and saline solution with a syringe or medicine dropper and place it into the nebulizer cup.

3. Attach the T-piece and the mouth piece to the cup or attach the mask to the cup. Attach the cup to the air compressor with the plastic tubing.

4. Plug the compressor into an outlet and turn it on.

5. Place the mouth piece in the child's mouth or place the mask over the child's face. Tell the child to breathe slowly and deeply (▼ **Figure 13-4**). The child should continue breathing the mist until the cup is empty, about 10 minutes.

Cleaning and Care of a Nebulizer

A child care provider should be trained to clean and care for each individual machine, based on the manufacturer's recommendations, because these machines can vary.

1. After each use, disassemble all parts of the nebulizer and put the plastic tubing aside. Clean the plastic mouth piece, the T-shaped piece or the mask, and the nebulizer cup with mild soap and warm water; let them air dry (▼ **Figures 13-5 and 13-6**).

2. Reassemble the unit, connect the tubing, and allow it to run for 15 to 20 seconds to complete the drying process.

3. Disconnect the tubing and store the plastic pieces in a clean container.

4. Wash the compressor only when it is disconnected. Use a disinfectant solution and a damp, clean cloth. Do not submerge the machine in water. When it is not in use, the compressor should be kept covered.

5. Change the air filter as needed.

6. Return the nebulizer to the child's parent at the end of each day for a thorough cleaning.

7. Keep a nebulizer and its medication out of the reach of children.

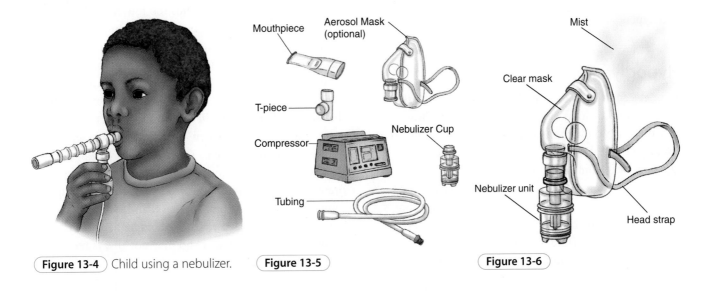

Figure 13-4 Child using a nebulizer.   **Figure 13-5**   **Figure 13-6**

Managing Asthma with Medication

Asthma is managed with 2 different types of medications—the *regulators* and the *rescuers*. Regulators are medicines that work to keep asthma under control and prevent asthma attacks. Rescuers are medicines that work to relieve acute asthma attacks. It is important to know if a child's medication is a regulator or a rescuer.

It is routine for children with asthma to take regulator medicines. These are usually in the form of a capsule, liquid, or powder that is taken by mouth 1 or more times each day. When a child's asthma symptoms are minimized or controlled, the child can be typically active and have lung function as near normal as possible. In addition, a child whose asthma is well-regulated has a reduced risk of medication side effects. Common side effects of the regulator medicines include dizziness, headache, and nausea. Medications prescribed as regulators need to be given regularly and on time.

When an acute asthma attack occurs, it is treated with a rescuer medication, usually from an inhaler or a nebulizer. An inhaler is a hand-held spray device that releases a powder or mist that the child can breathe deeply into the lungs. This medication relieves muscle spasms in the airway and makes breathing easier within several minutes.

Although the use of an inhaler might appear simple, it is often difficult for a young child to coordinate releasing the mist with inhaling. This is why an inhaler is often used with a spacer, or a holding chamber. This plastic attachment ensures the delivery of an even puff of medicine and prevents the medicine from being deposited on the tongue or on the back of the throat. A holding chamber is recommended for use with steroid medicines but not for dry powder medicines.

A nebulizer is a medical device that dispenses liquid medicine in the form of a mist through a mouth piece or a mask. It is most often used to deliver medication to very young children who are unable to use an inhaler.

Common side effects of rescuer medicines include nervousness, shakiness, and a feeling that the heart is beating rapidly. These side effects should pass within 15 to 20 minutes. Never give more medicine than is prescribed by the child's health care provider because this could increase the side effects.

All asthma medications should be kept at room temperature and away from direct sunlight. Excessive heat or refrigeration can alter the gas propellant in the medication container, resulting in delivery of an incorrect dose. Keep all asthma medicines out of the reach of children.

Diabetic Emergencies

Diabetes is a chronic illness that affects both adults and children and interferes with their ability to produce insulin and regulate blood sugar. Uncontrolled diabetes can produce two separate medical crises: hypoglycemia and hyperglycemia.

Hypoglycemia

Hypoglycemia is an abnormally low level of glucose, or sugar, in the blood. In the diabetic child, it means that there is too much insulin and not enough glucose circulating in the bloodstream. This causes an insulin reaction, or insulin shock, which comes on quickly and must be treated immediately. It is the most common medical emergency for a child with diabetes and can be life-threatening if ignored.

In a nondiabetic child, insulin levels rise and fall automatically in response to meals and activity levels.

But children with diabetes cannot produce insulin, so they must receive 1 or 2 insulin injections each day. They must also regulate their meals and activities so that there is always enough glucose in the blood to balance the amount of insulin.

If the blood glucose level dips too low, hypoglycemia occurs. This can happen if the child does not eat enough food, waits too long for a snack or meal, is unusually physically active, or receives too much insulin.

For a diabetic child, an important part of controlling the disease is learning to recognize the early sensations that signal when an insulin reaction is about to happen. A trained child knows when a reaction can happen, knows how to recognize its onset, and knows what to do. Immediately consuming a piece of candy, a glass of orange juice, or another quick source of sugar will rapidly return blood sugar to a proper level and avoid the insulin reaction altogether. However, a young diabetic child or a newly diagnosed diabetic child may not always recognize these signs early enough.

What To Look For

Early signs (which appear suddenly):

- Hunger
- Anger, irritability
- Weakness
- Trembling
- Sweating
- Dizziness

Later signs:

- Drowsiness
- Impaired thinking and coordination
- Confusion
- Loss of consciousness

What to Do

1. Give the child a fast-acting sugar, such as table sugar, a sugar cube, honey, cake frosting, candy, or orange juice, if the child is alert enough to swallow. The child should feel better in 10 to 15 minutes. Check whether the child missed a meal or snack.

2. If there is no improvement in 15 minutes, give the same amount of sugar again and call the child's parent or health care provider.

Caution:

DO NOT give the child a diet soft drink, because it does not contain any sugar.

DO NOT give sugar in a liquid form, such as juice or a soft drink, to an unconscious diabetic child.

Hyperglycemia

Hyperglycemia occurs when there is too much glucose and not enough insulin in the bloodstream. Persistent high blood sugar levels impair circulation, damage blood vessels and organs, and make the child particularly susceptible to infection.

Hyperglycemia occurs in a child with an undiagnosed case of diabetes. It can also occur in a child who has diabetes; when it does, it indicates either an illness or a need to readjust insulin dose or food intake. Hyperglycemia is not an immediate medical emergency in terms of first aid. It can take several days or even weeks to recognize the signs and symptoms.

What to Look For

- Excessive thirst
- Excessive hunger
- Sudden unexplained weight loss
- Fruity breath odor
- Excessive urination
- Weakness

A child who does not have diabetes can show one or two of these symptoms occasionally. But a child with developing or poorly controlled diabetes will persistently show several of these signs.

What to Do

If a child consistently has some of the above signs and symptoms, he or she should be seen by a health care provider. Untreated hyperglycemia results in further deterioration of the child's health.

HIV in a Child Care Setting

HIV (human immunodeficiency virus) is one of the largest health problems that the world faces today. The Centers for Disease Control estimates that in the United States alone, more than 1 million people are infected with HIV, which causes AIDS (acquired immune deficiency syndrome). Initially, HIV lives within the body for months or years before the signs and symptoms of AIDS appear. In time, the virus begins to destroy the immune system, making the body susceptible to chronic infections that become increasingly difficult to fight. Illnesses such as chicken pox and flu that might be minor to a person with a healthy immune system can be dangerous and even life-threatening to a person with HIV.

People who have HIV in their blood but have a healthy immune system are able to fight infection. Healthy HIV-infected persons can still transmit the virus to others, even though they have no symptoms of the disease and might not know they are infected. There is presently no vaccine or cure for HIV.

HIV is found in infected blood, semen, vaginal secretions, and breast milk. The virus is also present in other body fluids, including saliva, tears, perspiration, urine, and feces, but not in concentrations high enough to transmit the disease. However, the virus can be spread through any of these fluids if they contain HIV-infected blood, even in microscopic amounts.

HIV is a fragile virus and is not easily transmitted from person to person through ordinary, everyday activities. Some behaviors have been identified as high risk for transmitting HIV. These include unprotected sexual activity, sharing needles and syringes for drug use, body piercing and tattooing with uncleaned needles, sharing a toothbrush or a razor, and allowing blood or any body fluid containing even microscopic amounts of blood to come in contact with an open cut or sore, no matter how small the opening or where it is located.

HIV can be transmitted from an HIV-infected mother to her unborn child. Some children born to HIV-infected mothers initially test positive for HIV. Many of these

DIABETIC EMERGENCIES

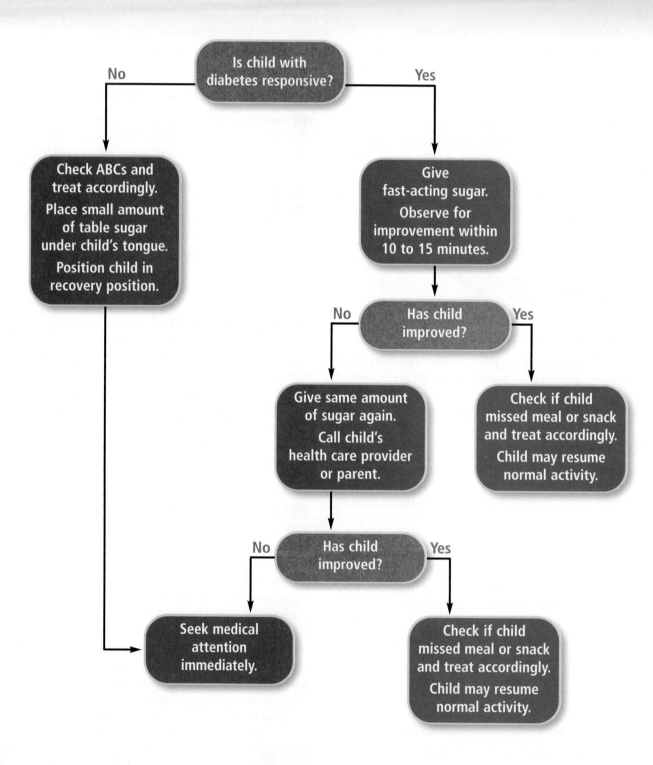

Diabetes Explained

During normal digestion, food is broken down into a sugar called glucose, which the body uses as fuel for the cells. Glucose enters the bloodstream, where it is transported from the blood into the cells with the help of insulin. The pancreas normally produces insulin whenever food is eaten and releases that insulin into the blood. The insulin then attaches to the glucose and transports it from the blood into the cells to nourish them. Without insulin, the glucose is available in the bloodstream but is unable to get to the cells. The cells do not get nourished, and the body begins to starve. This leads to weakness and fatigue. In addition, the high level of glucose in the bloodstream makes the body particularly susceptible to infection.

The accumulating glucose is filtered out of the blood by the kidneys and spills into the urine. This process requires extra water, which produces *thirst*. The glucose in the urine is lost, leaving the body unnourished, and producing insatiable *hunger*. The body turns to its supply of stored fat to make energy, which produces significant *weight loss*. These are the 3 telling signs of the development of diabetes—weight loss, thirst, and hunger.

Unlike glucose, fat does not require insulin for transport into the cells. However, in using fats for energy, the body produces unhealthy wastes called ketones. A buildup of ketones in the blood results in a condition known as ketoacidosis. If ketoacidosis is left untreated, it can lead to coma and death. The buildup of ketones in the blood produces *a fruity odor to the breath,* which is another indicator of developing diabetes.

Special Considerations for a Child with Diabetes

Diabetes is a lifelong illness that affects every aspect of the child's life. Constant daily insulin injections and blood tests for glucose, as well as lifelong dietary restrictions make diabetes a demanding disease.

The delicate balance between glucose and insulin levels in the blood is affected by the child's diet, physical activity, illness, and stress. Controlling the disease successfully in a child requires a team effort that involves the child, the parents, the health care provider, and the child care provider.

Diet. A child with diabetes needs foods that are high in nutritional value and low in concentrated sugar. It is essential for meals and snacks to be eaten at regular intervals to maintain the balance between glucose and insulin. Most children with diabetes need a morning and an afternoon snack. Parents should give providers specific instructions about their child's diet.

Parties and holiday celebrations present special problems when restricted foods are plentiful in the classroom. Occasionally, food exchanges and substitutions that allow a child to eat special treats are permitted but should be discussed with the child's parent.

Physical Activity. Most children with diabetes should be encouraged to participate fully in all activities of the child care center or school. Parents should provide information on any necessary restrictions. Strenuous activity can upset the balance between insulin and glucose in the blood and cause insulin shock. Do not restrict the child's activities for fear of insulin shock; instead, understand that the child's diet can be adjusted to ensure that the child has the additional energy necessary for energetic play or a special activity.

Illness and Stress. Illness and stress increase the demands on the body because they upset the balance between glucose and insulin. A provider must be especially watchful of a child with diabetes who is ill or stressed.

children, however, will lose the HIV antibody as they naturally lose other maternal antibodies during their first year of life. Therefore, a positive test for HIV shortly after birth is not a reliable indicator that the child actually is infected with HIV. In rare cases, HIV has been transmitted to a healthy infant by an HIV-infected mother through her breast milk.

HIV can also be transmitted through a transfusion of blood or blood products contaminated with the virus. However, this risk is very small because all blood and blood products are now carefully screened for HIV. There is no risk of becoming infected with HIV when donating blood.

HIV is *not* spread through such ordinary everyday activities as:

- Hugging
- Dry kissing
- Holding hands
- Sneezing or coughing
- Cooking
- Sharing foods
- Using public telephones
- Using public restrooms
- Using public swimming pools
- Touching money, furniture, doorknobs, etc.
- Using playground equipment and sandboxes
- Sharing books and toys
- Playing with a cat or a dog
- Being bitten by a mosquito
- Having an ear pierced by a commercial hand-held puncher

According to the U.S. Surgeon General's office, there are no documented cases of HIV transmission from one child to another in a school, child care, or foster care setting. Transmission of the virus in these settings would require the unlikely contact of one child's open cut with the blood or other body fluids of an HIV-infected child.

The number of children with HIV in child care in the United States is small but growing. However, for every child known to have HIV, there are other HIV-infected children whose health care providers, parents, and child care provider do not yet know that the virus is present. It is therefore essential for all child care providers to know how to handle body fluids correctly. Child care providers must:

- Wear disposable gloves when giving first aid for a cut or wound, changing diapers, and handling or wiping up body fluids such as blood and vomit. If gloves are not immediately available when first aid is necessary, use another barrier. Examples of

other barriers are several thick gauze pads, a clean dish towel, or a cloth diaper. Plastic wrap or a plastic bag placed over the gauze or cloth increases the effectiveness of these barriers.

- Use disposable diapers. Soiled diapers should be folded with the soiled side inward and placed in a double-lined, covered diaper pail.
- Clean blood and other fluids off all surfaces with a solution of 10 parts water to 1 part bleach. Allow this solution to air dry.
- Wash your hands vigorously with soap and warm water after removing disposable gloves.

Handle *all* body fluids for *all* children in this manner at *all* times.

Information contained in a child's medical record is confidential. A child care center must protect the privacy of a child who is infected with HIV by limiting the number of people who have knowledge of the child's condition. Each case of a child with HIV in a child care setting must be evaluated individually to determine how the center can best provide for the needs of the child. Decisions should be made jointly by the child's parent, health care provider, and child care center director and should be reevaluated periodically.

The problem of HIV infections and AIDS in the United States is growing at an alarming rate and child care providers continue to see increasing numbers of children with HIV. Child care providers must take responsibility for keeping up with new information on HIV and AIDS. Contact your local public health department or state AIDS information office, or call the National AIDS Information Hot Line (toll free): 1-800-342-AIDS. Spanish-speaking persons can call Linea Nacional de SIDA (toll free): 1-800-344-SIDA.

Children with Developmental and Medical Disabilities

Today children who have disabilities are educated in general education classrooms in neighborhood schools alongside children without disabilities. This kind of interaction is often termed inclusion or integration. Significant data, as well as thousands of anecdotal stories, demonstrate success for all students by including those with disabilities along with their nondisabled friends. In addition, children whose conditions require the care of a nurse are also finding a place in general education classrooms. Examples of such children, termed "medically fragile," include children who may have a tracheostomy, a feeding tube, a need for oxygen, an impaired immune system, or a life-threatening illness.

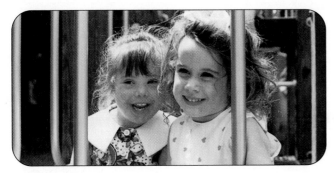

Figure 13-7 Child care centers and schools are now integrated.

It is hoped that typical children who are accustomed to being with children with disabilities as a natural part of school life will not have the misconceptions that people with disabilites are inferior, unapproachable, and nothing like them. After all, any individual or child could become disabled or seriously ill, either temporarily or permanently, at any time (▲ **Figure 13-7**).

Advocates for children who have disabilities feel that this type of education is the next step in breaking down social barriers in a civilized society. This is more than just the right thing to do; the law also requires that these children have a place in general education classrooms that meets their unique needs. The Education of the Handicapped Act, Public Law 94-142, was passed by Congress in 1975, amended in 1986, and amended again in 1990. At that time, it became know as IDEA, which stands for Individuals with Disabilities Education Act. A free public education is a right, not a privilege, for all Americans, and those who have a disability are not to be discounted.

Beginning at the age of 3, all children with disabilities must receive services from state agencies and school systems. Infants and toddlers are also covered by an early intervention component of the law. This identifies children from birth to age 3 who are experiencing developmental delays and provides support and services for them and their families to assist in their development.

The inclusion of preschool children who have disabilities in typical child care centers and nursery schools is the beginning of the educational and social experience for these children. In many of today's child care centers and nursery schools, there are children who use wheelchairs, walkers, and other adaptive equipment, children with visual and hearing impairments, and children who have a myriad of medical problems, developmental delays, and behavioral disabilities. To adequately support them in the child care or school setting, children with disabilities might also receive services from special education teachers or teaching assistants, nurses, physical therapists, occupational therapists, adaptive physical therapists, or speech therapists.

Children with special needs should be treated like other children as much as possible. Being held to many of the same standards as the other children in their class helps them gain self-confidence and independence. It also helps to correct some of the inaccurate assumptions that adults and other children sometimes make about them and their capabilities.

As a child care provider, you might sometimes feel frustrated and even sad for the child's situation, but it is important not to feel pity. Allowing yourself to feel pity lowers your expectations for the child; this lowered set of standards can be recognized by the child and negatively affect progress and overall success. As you get to know the child, you learn where the child's strengths lie. Expecting the child to conform to as many rules as possible, participate with the others, and attempt new experiences helps him or her have a positive preschool experience. A child with a disability is often a happy child who does not live in a constant state of frustration, is often just as healthy overall as a typical child, and feels all the same emotions as other children.

Generally, when a child with special needs attends a child care center, the center's staff receives instructions about special circumstances that might need attention, such as toileting, eating, or special precautions concerning outdoor play activities. In many instances, you need to make special arrangements or adaptations to help the child participate. Professional therapists often involve center staff in therapy sessions and encourage typical children to be part of group sessions that promote activities with peers in conjunction with the benefits of the particular therapy.

Often, parents are strong advocates for their children. They are usually your best resource for discovering the child's strengths and needs and for finding activities that can challenge the child and help the child excel. They can help you determine how best to include the child in a circle of friends within the child care center.

Nondisabled children in the child care center adjust easily to having a friend with a special need. Young children do not have opinions or prejudices concerning disabilities, only healthy curiosity. Children at this age do not hesitate to speak what is on their minds, and they ask simple questions that can be answered fairly easily. If their questions are answered in a matter-of-fact way, the friendship between them and the disabled child will develop naturally. Young children should be encouraged to ask questions about disabilities and should never be made to feel embarrassed or wrong for asking a question. Questions like, "Why are you in a wheelchair?" "Why do you wear a helmet?" "Why does that lady come to see you?" or "Why can't he walk to the play yard by himself?" are common and demonstrate that children are paying attention to their environment and noticing, but not condemning, differences. Straightforward answers that do not reveal your own biases or frustrations are your best response.

Learning Activities

Children With Medical Conditions That Affect Child Care

Directions: Circle Yes if you agree with the statement, and circle No if you disagree.

Yes   No   **1.** Hypoglycemia is the most common type of diabetic emergency.

Yes   No   **2.** It is important to offer fluids to a child having an asthma attack.

Yes   No   **3.** Air pollution, exercise, and cold weather can stimulate an asthma attack.

Yes   No   **4.** The incidence of asthma is on the decline due to more effective medicines.

Yes   No   **5.** During an asthma attack, the breathing passages relax, making it hard to clear mucus.

Yes   No   **6.** A standard asthma care plan is generally adequate for all children with asthma.

Yes   No   **7.** A child with hypoglycemia has too much glucose and not enough insulin.

Yes   No   **8.** Consuming a source of sugar, such as candy or orange juice, can help with hypoglycemia.

Yes   No   **9.** Signs of hypoglycemia include excessive thirst, hunger, and fruity breath odor.

Yes   No   **10.** HIV can live in the human body for months or years before symptoms of AIDS appear.

Yes   No   **11.** HIV is easily transmitted through ordinary activities such as sneezing or hugging.

Yes   No   **12.** Young children should be discouraged from asking classmates with disabilities direct questions about their conditions.

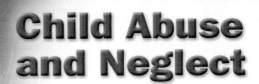

Chapter 14

Child Abuse and Neglect

Child abuse and neglect are tragic problems that cause suffering and fear for thousands of children. Child abuse is defined as physical injury, emotional mistreatment, neglect, or sexual abuse that is willfully inflicted on a child. Many children die each year from injuries inflicted by abusive adults. Many more survive years of these abuses and suffer permanent physical, developmental, and psychological damage. An abused child often has low self-esteem and difficulty relating to others.

Child abuse and neglect occur at all levels of society and in all cultures. It is a very old problem that was quietly tolerated by society until recently. Fortunately, significant public and professional attention has forced society to pay attention to a problem that jeopardizes the health and future of so many children.

Child care providers are trusted figures to young children. Your regular interaction with a small group of children allows you to observe closely a child's conduct and appearance and to notice clues that might indicate a risk to the child's health and safety at home or elsewhere.

Today, children are exposed to a variety of adult authority figures such as teachers, child care providers, parents, other relatives, parents' significant others, and teenage baby sitters. Children need to feel safe in the company of every adult who cares for them.

Physical Abuse

Physical abuse is a willful act of cruelty or violence against a child that results in an injury. It is often the result of unjustified or severe punishment and can occur when the adult is angry or frustrated and becomes violent toward the child with behaviors such as hitting, shaking, biting, throwing the child, or twisting a limb. Some abusive acts such as burning or beating with a belt are deliberate and premeditated. Often, physical abuse is a chronic situation. Frequent unexplained or poorly explained injuries or an injury that is unusual for the child's age, such as a fracture in an infant, should raise concern. Also of concern are injuries whose descriptions do not seem plausible in light of the diagnosis from a health care provider.

What to Look For

Indications of possible child abuse in the child's appearance include:

- Head injuries are the most common cause of death from child abuse. Neurologic damage to the brain from a blow or from shaking can sometimes go undetected until pronounced symptoms develop, especially if there are no obvious signs of damage to the head or face.

- Scald burns are the most commonly inflicted burn injury. Some scalds result from hot liquids being thrown. Immersion burns look like a glove on the hand or a sock on the foot. Normally children withdraw immediately from pain, so that a well-defined margin on a burn, like a mark around the ankle or wrist from the level of hot water, is suspicious. Pattern or branding burns are the shape of the item used such as a cigarette or an iron, or a doughnut shape on the buttock from the burner of an electric stove.

- Burns from rope appear around the wrists or ankles if the child has been tied up.

- Bruises or welts can be located on hidden or visible areas of the body. Bruises on the buttocks, back, face, or genitals, or small paired bruises from forceful pinching are all common.

- Broken bone injuries may also indicate abuse, especially those that occur more than once or those in which the appearance of the injury does not match the description of how it happened.

- Lacerations, especially on the face from a hand, a foot, or from the impact of a heavy object.

- Bite marks appear as doughnut-shaped or double-horseshoe-shaped and may be discolored from bruising. In some bite marks, the tooth impressions help identify the biter, if they are shown to a health care provider promptly.

- Injuries in the mouth of an infant might indicate excessively forceful feeding.

Indications of possible child abuse in the child's behavior include:

- Becomes apprehensive when other children cry

- Appears afraid and hesitant to go with the abusive adult

- Is not trusting of physical contact with adults in the child care center

- Shows extremes of behavior from aggressiveness to isolation

- Might tell the child care provider what happened

Emotional Abuse

Emotional abuse is continual verbal degradation and insults that cause the child to feel worthless and empty. It can damage the child intellectually, behaviorally, and psychologically. A parent's distorted view of parenting, harsh or inconsistent reactions to family life events, and verbal violence can create emotional problems that continue to affect the child later in life. Often emotional abuse accompanies physical abuse. Domestic violence witnessed by a child is also considered to be emotional abuse. If the child is repeatedly degraded over a long time, the child will begin to believe that what is communicated by the abuser is true. Unfortunately, emotional abuse is very difficult to prove.

What to Look For

Indications of possible emotional abuse in the child's appearance include:

- Signs of physical abuse

- Failure to thrive, described as abnormally low weight in conjunction with abnormally slow development for no apparent medical reason

Indications of possible emotional abuse in the child's behavior include:

- Lags behind in intellectual, physical, and emotional development

Shaken Baby Syndrome

A severe degree of head injury can be inflicted on an infant who is roughly or violently shaken. Termed "shaken baby syndrome" or "shaken infant syndrome," it almost always occurs when a parent or other care giver shakes a crying baby in frustration, either to punish or to quiet the child. In most cases, it is the result of the adult losing self-control.

The infant's body proportions are very different from the adult's. Most significantly, the infant's head is oversized in comparison to the rest of the body, and the neck muscles are not strong enough to support the head during rough handling. Shaking an infant causes the head to flop back and forth, bruising the brain as it bangs against the skull wall.

This forceful shaking can result in bleeding, swelling, and pressure in the brain, damage to the eyes, injuries to the neck and spine, and sometimes death. Often there are no outward signs of trauma to the body. The child who survives this injury can be left with a seizure disorder, severe visual impairment, some degree of paralysis, or mental retardation. Incidents of less violent shaking often leave the child with learning disabilities.

In rare instances, these injuries result accidentally from a parent or other adult tossing the infant in the air as an act of affection or play or from jogging with an infant in a backpack.

To prevent the devastating effects of shaken baby syndrome:

+ Never shake an infant either in play or in anger.

+ Call someone to stay with the infant or place the infant in a safe location, such as in the crib, and walk away if you feel out of control.

+ Seek help from your local child abuse hotline for yourself or other care givers whose anger toward an infant causes you concern.

- Seems withdrawn and depressed

- Fluctuates emotionally between being unusually compliant and passive and being extremely aggressive, demanding, or violent

- Shows unusual adaptive behaviors, such as being inappropriately adult (for instance, parenting other children) or inappropriately infantile (for example, thumb sucking, frequent rocking, and urinary incontinence)

- Is considered a behavior problem, showing self-destructive behavior that might eventually lead to suicide attempts

- Makes statements such as, "Daddy says I'm a very bad boy"

Sexual Abuse

Sexual abuse consists of inappropriate physical contact with a child. This covers a wide range of crimes from fondling and indecent exposure to violent activities such as rape. Most cases of sexual abuse are recurrent and the child knows the sexual offender. The child might be sworn to secrecy by an abuser who has bribed the child or threatened violence or death to the child or another loved one if the child tells anyone.

What to Look For

Indications of possible sexual abuse in the child's appearance include:

- Irritation, pain, bruises, or bleeding in the genital area

- Discharge from the vagina or penis that could be from a sexually transmitted disease

- Stained or bloody underwear

Indications of possible sexual abuse in the child's behavior include:

- Has poor relationships with peers and withdraws from social activities

- Engages in abnormal fantasy or infantile behavior

- Has recurrent nightmares that might be shared with child care staff

- Has a greater conversational knowledge of sexual matters than is appropriate for his or her age

- Has inappropriate and excessive curiosity about sexual matters or private body parts of others

- Shows fear or hesitancy about going with a particular person

- Exhibits regressive behavior (in school-aged children), such as thumb sucking, excessive crying, and withdrawal into a fantasy world

- Engages in other inappropriate behaviors (in school-aged children), including aggressive or disruptive acting out, running away, delinquent activities, and failing in school work

- Might report incidents indirectly, such as, "I know someone who . . ." or "What would you do if . . . ?"

- Has problems with pants-wetting and fecal soiling

Neglect

A chronically neglected child suffers from a lack of care and protection, which can have an injurious effect on physical and emotional health. These children suffer from inadequate nutrition, clothing, shelter, personal and household hygiene, and medical care. Too often they lack proper supervision. They also lack consistent contact with nurturing and supportive adults outside of the child care setting. Children who are neglected in these ways are vulnerable to disease, injury, and a variety of social problems.

What to Look For

Indications of possible neglect in the child's appearance include:

- Has untreated medical problems and rarely sees a health care provider or a dentist for well-child care

- Looks unkempt, is inadequately dressed—especially in cold weather, looks and smells dirty, and has chronic mouth odor

- Conversation reveals that the child is often alone, cared for by another child, or engages in activities that are dangerous or inappropriate for his or her age

- Conversation causes you to suspect that home is unsanitary or lacks adequate heating or plumbing

Indications of possible neglect in the child's behavior include:

- Little experience with rules and limit-setting

- Behavior might appear delinquent compared with behavior of other children in the center or school

- Frequent use of foul language, which can indicate inappropriate language by adults or older children to whom the child is exposed outside of the child care center

- Frequent complaints of hunger and sneaking of food

- Often tired and lacks enthusiasm

- Has a poor attendance record with unexplained absences

How to Help

All adults need to be aware of the devastation that abuse in any form brings upon a child and must be willing to get involved. Child care providers and teachers are, in many states, defined as professionals who are required by law to report suspected child abuse to the state's protective services.

Some child care providers worry about hurting a trusted relationship with a young child by breaking confidentiality. It is important to report suspected abuse when you first become suspicious, because abuse is more often a pattern than a one-time incident and is likely to continue or even intensify. It is important not to tell the child that you will keep this shared information a secret, but rather to let the child know that you can help. You are a key person in recognizing the signs of child abuse and getting the system working to rescue a child from an abusive situation or to find services and support to help heal a dysfunctional family. For more information about how to help a child when abuse is suspected, call the National Child Abuse Hotline at 1-800-422-4453.

Learning Activities

Child Abuse and Neglect

Directions: Circle Yes if you agree with the statement, and circle No if you disagree.

Yes   No   **1.** Child abuse occurs at all levels of society and in all cultures.

Yes   No   **2.** Physical abuse is usually a one-time occurrence.

Yes   No   **3.** The infant's head muscles are not strong enough to support the head during rough handling.

Yes   No   **4.** As a child care provider, you are encouraged but not required by law to report suspected child abuse.

Chapter 15

Illness and Infection Prevention

Some children are the picture of health no matter what the season. Other children seem to pick up every illness to which they are exposed. On the average, toddlers and preschoolers experience 6 to 8 episodes of illness each year. This frequency decreases to about 3 episodes each year by the time a child is 6 years old. Fortunately, the incidence of many of the serious and life-threatening childhood illnesses has been dramatically reduced by vaccines and antibiotics. Today in the United States, common illnesses are generally mild compared to those of past generations.

What Causes Illness?

Viral infections include illnesses such as chicken pox, colds, croup, some pneumonias, and the gastrointestinal upsets of vomiting and diarrhea. Symptoms such as cough, congestion, and fever can be treated to make the child feel more comfortable. Pharmaceutical companies are working to develop medications to treat viral infections, but there are no effective medications available yet. Antibiotics have no effect on viruses. Most illness caused by viruses subside with time.

The viruses that cause the common cold, as well as many of the common upper respiratory infections, enter through the eyes, nose, and mouth. They are spread from one person to another as air-borne particles from a cough or a sneeze or by direct contact. If children sneeze into their hands and then pick up toys or touch a door knob without first washing their hands, they will contaminate these items with the virus.

Bacterial infections, which include illnesses such as ear infections, strep throat, scarlet fever, impetigo, and some pneumonias, must be treated by prescription antibiotics to ensure prompt and complete recovery. To help prevent an infection from recurring, it is important for a child taking an antibiotic to complete the entire course of medicine.

Fungal infections include such conditions as ringworm, athlete's foot, and thrush; they are usually not serious. There are several medications for fungal infections. Antibiotics are not prescribed to treat fungal infections and, in some instances, can worsen the condition.

Intestinal **parasitic infections** such as pinworms and giardia are common and are caused by worms and protozoa. They are transmitted by ingestion and need to be treated with a prescription medication specifically for the parasite.

How Illness Is Spread

Microorganisms that cause illness enter the body in one of these four ways:

- **Direct contact** or touching, as with the impetigo bacteria, the herpes virus, and the thrush fungus

- **Ingestion,** as with the pinworm parasite and the hepatitis A virus

- **Airborne transmission** of microorganisms through the eyes, nose, or mouth, as with the common cold, influenza, and chicken pox viruses or the strep throat bacteria

- **Blood to blood contact,** as with the HIV virus

Preventing Infection in a Child Care Setting

Spending many hours each day inside and in close contact with other youngsters invites the spread of illness. To decrease the incidence of illness among children in child care settings, providers must consistently practice good hygiene and encourage children to follow their example. All staff members should know and follow these good hygiene rules.

1. **Wash hands frequently.** This is the single most important measure to prevent the spread of illness and infection (▼ Figure 15-1).

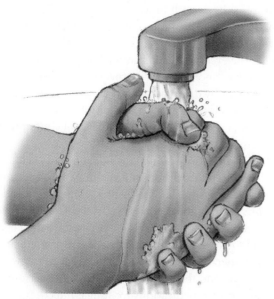

Figure 15-1 Hand washing with soap and warm water can help stop the spread of disease.

How to wash hands:

- Use liquid soap and warm water to scrub hands vigorously for 15 to 30 seconds. The friction created by rubbing the hands together contributes as much to the cleaning as does the soap and water. Wash the backs of the hands and under the fingernails.

- Rinse hands with warm running water and dry them with a paper towel. Then use the towel to turn off the faucet.

- Keep fingernails short and scrub with a nail brush. Organisms collect easily under long fingernails.

When to wash hands:

- Before eating or preparing foods

- After toileting, helping a child with toileting, or diapering

- After touching body fluids (saliva, nasal discharge, blood, tears, stool, urine) and after removing disposable gloves

When to have children wash their hands:

- After toileting. Young children need to be taught, reminded, and supervised. Infants and toddlers who wear diapers should have their hands washed after diaper changes if they touch the diaper area.

- After playing outside

- Before participating in a cooking project

- Before meal and snack times

- Before playing with play dough

2. **Disinfect all washable surfaces.** Use a commercial disinfectant or a sanitizing solution of bleach and water. The solution should be made of 1 part bleach to 10 parts water and must be made fresh daily. It is inexpensive and extremely effective in killing germs. Spray it on all washable surfaces and allow it to air dry. Disinfect the following surfaces daily:

- Sinks

- Toilets

- Potty seats

- Diaper changing tables

- Table tops

- Door knobs

Toys that the children put in their mouths should be washed daily, rinsed with the sanitizing solution, rinsed with water, and allowed to air dry.

Vomit, diarrhea, and blood should be wiped up with gloved hands, and the surface should be disinfected. Soiled clothing and bedding should be placed in a plastic bag and sent home.

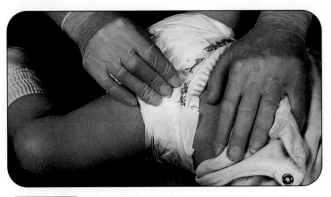

3. **Use disposable gloves.** Disposable gloves act as a barrier between your skin and another person's body fluids, such as blood, diarrhea, urine, and vomit. Gloves should be worn when there is a chance of touching these fluids, because of the many organisms they can contain that transmit disease. Gloves also protect a child with an open wound from contaminants on the provider's hands.

   Disposable gloves should be available in each bathroom, in the diaper changing area, and in the first aid kit (▲ **Figure 15-2**). Wash hands thoroughly with soap and water after removing disposable gloves. Throw the gloves away after one use.

4. **Practice good hygiene and encourage the children to follow your example.**
   • Tie long hair back.
   • Do not share personal items, such as brushes, hats, toothbrushes, cups, washcloths, and drinking straws.
   • Keep fingernails clean and trimmed.
   • Do not bite fingernails, rub eyes, or otherwise touch the face without washing hands first. Touching the face and mouth can introduce germs that cause colds and other illnesses. Cover your mouth when coughing and sneezing.
   • Discard used tissues promptly.
   • Spend part of every day outdoors.
   • Leave the doors and windows open while the children are outdoors, weather permitting, to circulate fresh air.
   • Make your center smoke-free.
   • Practice good hygiene routinely, not just when a child is ill.

5. **Maintain clean play areas.**
   • Drain wading pools daily and as needed. Drain, clean, and disinfect water tables daily and allow them to air dry. Clean and disinfect water toys.
   • Cover outside sandboxes so they do not become litter boxes. The ingestion of microscopic particles of animal waste can cause illness.
   • Put rubber pants over diapers, even disposable diapers, when taking a young child into a wading pool.
   • Lawn sprinklers are more hygienic than wading pools for water play.

6. **Handle and prepare foods properly.**
   • Wash hands before handling food. Be aware of what you touch during food preparation and rewash hands as necessary.
   • Tie hair back, or wear a hair net.
   • Do not handle food when you are ill.
   • Avoid changing diapers if you are a food preparer. In a home child care setting, where there is only one provider, good hand washing technique is essential.
   • Keep the diaper-changing area separate from the food area.
   • Do not taste the food with a utensil that is used to cook and stir.
   • Use separate surfaces and utensils when preparing meat.
   • Wash all dishes and eating utensils in an automatic dishwasher with the booster thermostat set to 170°F (76.6°C). If a dishwasher is unavailable, wash dishes and utensils with hot water and soap, rinse in a sanitizing solution of bleach (10 parts water to 1 part bleach), rinse again with clear water, and allow to air dry. If your center does not have proper cleaning facilities, disposable dishes and utensils must be used and then discarded.

7. **Take special precautions with infants.**
   • Wash mouthed toys daily with hot water and soap, rinse in a sanitizing solution of bleach (10 parts water to 1 part bleach), rinse again with water, and air dry.
   • Rinse a pacifier or a toy that was dropped on the floor before handing it back.
   • Wear a disposable or cloth gown when holding an infant under 6 months of age. Use a separate gown for each infant.

Many states have specific written requirements concerning infection control in a child care center. In addition, many centers have their own written guidelines, which were developed or approved by a health care consultant. Your center's staff should know your state guidelines.

Learning Activities

Illness and Infection Prevention

Directions: Circle Yes if you agree with the statement, and circle No if you disagree.

Yes   No   **1.** The common cold is caused by bacteria.

Yes   No   **2.** Antibiotics have no effect on bacterial illnesses.

Yes   No   **3.** Washing the hands is the single most important measure for controlling the spread of illness.

Yes   No   **4.** Practicing good hygiene is important only when a child is ill.

Yes   No   **5.** When washing hands, rubbing the hands together vigorously is as important as the soap and water.

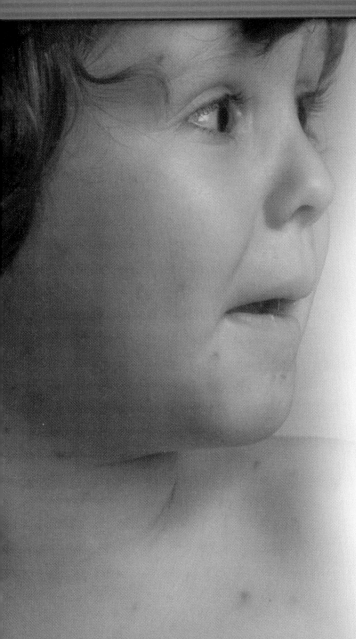

Chapter 16

Common Childhood Illnesses

Many bouts of childhood illnesses are caused by common viruses and are destroyed by the child's immune system in a matter of days. Some viral illnesses are more persistent, and the child takes longer to bounce back. A sick child should be monitored by a parent or provider to be sure that the child stays on the road to recovery or to seek care immediately if a complication develops.

Colds, diarrhea, fever, and vomiting are four common ailments that are actually symptoms of an infection. Usually, these infections are caused by viruses and, less often, by bacteria. These common ailments recur a number of times in young children. They occur year round but more often during the fall and winter months when colder temperatures and inclement weather keep windows closed and people close together. With children coughing in the enclosed space of a child care center, viral infections spread easily (**Figure 16-1 ▶**). Because the breeze blowing through the building clears the air by diluting the concentration of infective organisms, leave doors and windows open for a few minutes each day.

Colds

By far the most common ailment of young children is the common cold, which is caused by viruses and must run its course. Symptoms, including a runny or stuffy nose, sore throat, and cough, can last from 4 days to 2 weeks. A child might also have a fever during a cold, particularly at the beginning, as well as a headache and temporarily decreased appetite. "Not acting like herself" is often the best indicator of how sick the child feels. Most colds are not serious. The chief problem for child care providers and parents is keeping the child comfortable and the symptoms under control.

What to Do

- Use over-the-counter decongestants and cough medicines as recommended by the child's health care provider.

- Use a cool-mist vaporizer to reduce congestion and thin mucus. The vaporizer must be cleaned daily with soap and water, then rinsed with a solution of one part bleach to ten parts water.

- Use a nasal aspirator (suction bulb) for infants. To use, press the bulb flat and hold the tip at the opening or just inside the nostril; release and remove. This is especially helpful before meals and at naptime.

- The parent should call the child's health care provider if the child develops a fever or complains of pain in the ear, if the nasal drainage becomes yellow or green, or if the eyes develop a discharge or become crusty.

Trying to teach toddlers or preschoolers to blow the nose can be tricky. Children eventually develop this ability but it is hard to understand before the child is ready for it. If the child is too young, it is likely that the child will suck in rather than blow out, which only leads to further mucus congestion. When the child is ready to learn to blow the nose, try suggesting that the child think of blowing out birthday candles through the nose. This helps to start the purposeful exhalation necessary for success.

Diarrhea

When a child has diarrhea, the bowel movements, or stools, are loose (either mushy or very watery) and more frequent than is normal for the child. Sometimes diarrhea is accompanied by vomiting, stomach pain, or fever. Common causes are viral illnesses, antibiotic treatment (which upsets the balance of normal bacteria in the intestines), or diet (either a particular food or the quantity of a food). Less common causes include certain illnesses or bacterial or parasitic infections. See *Infectious Diarrhea* in the Common Childhood Illnesses chart.

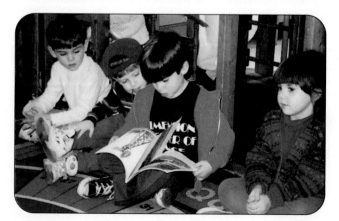

Figure 16-1 Viral infections can spread easily in the enclosed space of a child care center.

Most diarrhea resolves without treatment within a few days. Treating diarrhea involves giving the bowel a rest while making sure the child has enough fluid to replace what is lost in the stools. A young child with infectious diarrhea or diarrhea that cannot be contained should be kept at home until the necessary treatment is completed and negative results are obtained on stool cultures. Diarrhea is especially worrisome in infants, because a very small body can become dehydrated easily. See *Dehydration* in Chapter 12.

What to Do

1. **Give fluids.** During an acute episode of diarrhea, do not give solid food, but encourage small sips of clear fluids (fluids you can see through). Good choices for clear fluids are a pediatric electrolyte solution (available in grocery and drug stores) and a diluted sports or fruit drink. Clear fluids alone should not be given for more than 24 hours.

   For infants: If breastfeeding, continue and offer a pediatric electrolyte solution between feedings. If formula feeding, temporarily discontinue formula and give the pediatric electrolyte solution. If this solution is not available, give gelatin water made with twice as much water. Clear fluids alone should not be given for more than 24 hours.

When Diarrhea Becomes Worrisome

The parent should call the child's health care provider if:

+ the child is an infant under 6 months of age.

+ the child is unable to drink.

+ the child shows any signs of dehydration, such as dry lips and mouth, listlessness, no tears when crying, a dry diaper for several hours, or infrequent, small amounts of deep gold urine.

+ the child complains of severe abdominal pain.

+ there is blood, pus, or mucus in the stool.

+ diarrhea has not improved at all in 24 hours.

+ mild or moderate diarrhea persists longer than 1 week.

+ the child's diarrhea appears to be related to the use of an antibiotic.

2. **Provide good skin care.** Change diapers immediately and wash the skin after each diarrhea episode. Petroleum jelly creates a moisture barrier for the skin. Skin irritation caused by diarrhea may be so uncomfortable that even toilet-trained children complain of a burning sensation around the anus. Wash your hands after every diaper change or toileting assistance because diarrhea can be contagious.

3. **Slowly return to a regular diet.** Once the diarrhea begins to improve, slowly begin to offer foods that bind and slow the passage of stool through the intestines, such as bananas, applesauce, white toast without butter or margarine, crackers, rice cakes, dry cereals, noodles, rice, and other low-fat, bland foods. Continue to encourage the child to drink fluids. Temporarily avoid milk products and other fruits. Slowly return the child to a regular diet. Return milk, cheese, and ice cream to the diet last because they are difficult to digest.

   For infants: Offer applesauce, bananas, carrots, and rice cereal to infants on solid food. Slowly return to full-strength formula or offer a soy formula for several days, because it is more easily digested than a milk formula.

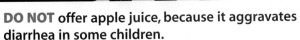

Caution:

DO NOT offer apple juice, because it aggravates diarrhea in some children.

Fever

Fever is an elevated temperature and is common in young children. The arrival of a fever triggers a period of discomfort and illness for the child and concern for the parents. A fever is not an illness; it is a symptom of an illness. It is not harmful and, in fact, is beneficial in fighting an illness. However, a prolonged fever can be of concern when the illness responsible for it is not diagnosed and treated.

Why does a child get a fever? When the body's defense system, known as the immune system, finds an invading organism such as a bacteria or a virus, certain "fighter" blood cells surround the invader to destroy it. This triggers a message to the brain to "turn up the heat." The higher body temperature created by the fever helps the fighter cells because they work more effectively at above-normal temperatures. A fever is worrisome in a child under the age of 6 months, because a young infant cannot fight infection as easily as older children and can more easily become dehydrated.

The normal oral temperature reading is 98.6°F. During an illness, it is not unusual for a young child's fever to run as high as 105°F. A temperature can be measured orally, rectally, or under the arm (axillary) with a standard glass or digital thermometer, or in the ear (auricular) with a small probe that measures the infrared heat produced in the eardrum and surrounding tissue.

Readings will vary depending on where the temperature is taken. The method you use depends on the age of the child. Taking the temperature rectally gives the most accurate reading; however, it is unnecessarily intrusive to an older child. A rectal temperature reading registers 1 degree higher than an oral temperature reading. An axillary temperature reading registers 1°F lower than an oral reading.

A glass thermometer can take up to 1 minute to register rectally, 3 minutes to register orally, and 10 minutes to register under the arm. Some glass thermometers are designed for oral use and others for rectal use. A digital thermometer can be used to take either an oral, rectal, or axillary temperature and takes only 1 minute to register. An ear probe heat sensor takes only seconds to register and provides a reading comparable to an oral reading.

Taking an oral temperature is not recommended for children age 4 and under because they have not developed the ability to hold the thermometer under the tongue with the mouth closed. Avoid giving a cold drink prior to taking an oral temperature.

What to Do

Because a fever is not an illness in itself, it is not possible to "cure" the fever. A moderate fever (99°F to 102°F) can promote the body's infection-fighting system without causing discomfort to the child or worry to parents.

Recommended Methods for Taking Child's Temperature by Age

Age of Child	Rectal	Axillary	Oral	Auricular
1 year and younger	•	•		•
2 years		•		•
3 years		•		•
4 years		•		•
5 years and older		•	•	•

1. Separate the child from other children and notify the child's parent, because a fever is often associated with a contagious illness. The child should remain at home until fever-free for 24 hours or, if necessary, until examined by a health care provider.

2. Encourage sips of clear fluids (fluids you can see through), such as water, tea, "flat" ginger ale, finely crushed ice, popsicles, and gelatin. Apple juice is a clear fluid but it can cause diarrhea in some children and should be avoided.

3. Give acetaminophen if the fever is above 101°F. Give the recommended dosage prescribed by the child's health care provider. Know your center's policy on administering medication. A parent might find it helpful to have children's acetaminophen suppositories on hand. They are an easy way to get fever-reducing medicine into a child who is also nauseated, is vomiting, or is too ill to swallow liquid or pills. They can be purchased over-the-counter but are kept under refrigeration, so the parent must ask for them.

4. Dress the child as lightly as possible, but do not allow the child to shiver. Shivering closes the skin pores and can increase the body temperature. The child feels alternately hot and cold as the fever goes up and down.

5. Sponge bathe a child if the fever is over 103°F. Rub the skin briskly using tepid water (75°F to 85°F) and a face cloth. Do not use cold water. Keep the water warm enough so that the child does not shiver. Wet the head because almost half of the body's heat loss is through the head. As the water evaporates, it will help cool the body.

Caution:

DO NOT give aspirin or any product containing salicylate to a child with a fever unless a health care provider tells you to do so.

Vomiting

Nausea and vomiting are common symptoms of a stomach virus and should last no longer than 24 hours. A slight fever or diarrhea might accompany the nausea and vomiting. The obvious worry about vomiting is that it can lead to dehydration. A child who is vomiting should be moved away from other children.

What to Do

1. Give nothing to eat or drink until 1 hour after the child last vomited.

2. After 1 hour has passed, offer sips of water or ice chips every 15 to 20 minutes to keep the child adequately hydrated. Big gulps will likely result in more vomiting. Offer the child a wet face cloth to suck on to keep the mouth and lips moist. If the child begins to vomit again, allow the stomach to rest for another 30 minutes to 1 hour and then start over. If the child tolerates small sips of water for 1 hour, offer sips of other clear fluids such as tea, "flat" ginger ale (shaken until all bubbles are gone), a diluted sports or fruit drink, a pediatric electrolyte solution (available in grocery and drug stores), gelatin water made with twice as much water, or popsicles.

3. Wait several hours before offering food. Begin with foods that are easily tolerated such as rice cakes, dry cereal, dry toast, and crackers. Avoid offering solids and clear liquids together because they might cause the nausea or vomiting to return.
   For infants: Offer applesauce, bananas, and rice cereal. The child should be back on a regular diet within 1 to 2 days after the vomiting.

Caution:

DO NOT stop breast-feeding unless instructed to do so by your child's health care provider.

When Vomiting Becomes Worrisome

The parent should call the child's health care provider if:

+ the child is an infant under 6 months of age.

+ the child is unable to keep any fluid in the stomach for several hours.

+ the child shows signs of dehydration such as dry lips and mouth, listlessness, no tears, a dry diaper for several hours, or infrequent, small amounts of deep gold urine.

+ the child has severe abdominal pain.

+ vomiting is forceful and projectile.

+ there is blood in the vomit.

Common Childhood Illness Quick Reference

The following alphabetical chart of symptoms or health complaints that a child might describe provides information about several illnesses and health conditions commonly experienced by children. Each symptom provides recommendations helpful to child care providers and to parents, and many topics suggest common, but not all, diagnoses for the symptom.

Anal Itching

Possible Diagnosis: Pinworms

What You Should Know

- An intestinal parasitic worm infection.

- Acquired by ingesting microscopic pinworm eggs after outdoor play in dirt or sand.

- Common among young children who often have their hands in their mouths, and are poor hand washers.

- Can cause intense rectal/anal itching.

- Highly contagious in a family or child care setting.

- Spreads to others when child scratches anal area, getting eggs under fingernails, and then touches another's food or other items that might be mouthed. Also spreads from eggs on pajamas, linens, underpants, etc.

- Diagnosed with a special pinworm kit used by parent to collect parasite specimen from anal skin.

What You Can Do As a Caregiver

- Discourage scratching anal area.

- Encourage child to wash hands after outdoor play.

- Notify parent.

What You Can Do As a Parent

- Follow Caregiver recommendations.

- Trim the child's fingernails short.

- Wash child's bed linen, clothing, and towels in hot water and dry on high heat setting; do not shake items because this will scatter the eggs.

Child May Return to School or Child Care . . .

after child has been treated initially and after itching subsides.

Constipation

What You Should Know

- Defined as hard stools that cause painful elimination.

- Can be caused by diet low in fiber and inadequate fluid intake.

- Sometimes caused by postponing or resisting urge to eliminate.

What You Can Do As a Caregiver

- Encourage child to drink clear fluids.

- Encourage child to eat foods that contain fiber and have a tendency to soften the stool such as whole grains, peaches, prunes, grapes, raisins, plums, melons, carrots, celery, and lettuce.

- Reduce intake of foods that bind such as milk, hard cheese, cottage cheese, bananas, apples, applesauce, and white-flour baked goods.

- Encourage regular toileting.

What You Can Do As a Parent

- Follow Caregiver recommendations.

- Call child's health care provider if problem persists for several weeks.

Child May Return to School or Child Care . . .

Child need not be excluded from school or child care.

Common Childhood Illness Quick Reference

Coughing

What You Should Know

- A symptom of an irritation within the respiratory tract.
- Often accompanies a viral infection such as a cold.
- Also see *Croup* in Chapter 12.

What You Can Do As a Caregiver

- Encourage child to cover mouth when coughing and to wash hands thoroughly and often.
- See the section on *Colds* in this chapter, and *Preventing Infection in a Child Care Setting* in Chapter 15.

What You Can Do As a Parent

- Follow Caregiver recommendations.
- Notify child's health care provider if child develops a fever or if cough persists for longer than 1 week.

Child May Return to School or Child Care . . .

Child need not be excluded from school or child care unless cough is accompanied by fever.

Possible Diagnosis: Pertussis (Whooping Cough)

What You Should Know

- Commonly known as "whooping cough" because of the whooping noise a child makes when coughing.
- Highly contagious bacterial infection.
- Spreads to others through coughing and sneezing.
- Incubation period averages 7 to 10 days.
- Generally a mild illness in older children, but can be life-threatening to infants because of breathing difficulties, pneumonia, and brain swelling.
- First stage of infection lasts approximately 1 week and mimics the usual cold symptoms of runny nose, sneezing, and coughing, which can delay diagnosis.
- Second stage lasts approximately 4 to 6 weeks, with uncontrollable coughing spells, often accompanied by whooping noise when child inhales. Cough can be so violent that it causes vomiting. Child may cough up thick mucus.
- Diagnosed by nasal culture within first 2 weeks of coughing and with a blood test if cough has lasted longer than 2 weeks.
- Treated with antibiotics for 14 days.
- Vaccine is given to infants as part of DPT (diptheria, pertussis, tetanus) immunization to protect young children, but immunity diminishes as years pass.
- A pertussis infection gives lifelong immunity.
- Centers for Disease Control require all health care providers and state medical labs to report positive culture results for pertussis to the Department of Public Health.

What You Can Do As a Caregiver

- Encourage parent of a child with a prolonged cough to take the child to a health care provider.
- Alert other parents if a child is diagnosed with pertussis. Encourage them to contact their health care providers. Maintain confidentiality.
- For more information, contact your local Department of Public Health.

What You Can Do As a Parent

- Have child seen by health care provider for prolonged cough.

Child May Return to School or Child Care . . .

after the first 5 days of 14-day antibiotic treatment course.

Diaper Rash

Possible Diagnosis: Simple Diaper Rash

What You Should Know

- Commonly occurs when bacteria in bowel react with urine to form ammonia, which irritates and burns skin.

- Can worsen with prolonged exposure to soiled diapers and friction against skin.

- Can be painful.

What You Can Do As a Caregiver

- Change diapers often; wear disposable gloves.

- Wash diaper area with soap and warm water; allow to dry completely.

- Place child in cool baths with one half cup vinegar for 15 to 20 minutes, several times per day. Vinegar reduces bacterial growth and helps to neutralize ammonia.

- Protect diaper area with over-the-counter ointments such as zinc oxide or petroleum jelly, which act as moisture barriers.

- Wash hands thoroughly after removing gloves.

- Do not use baby powder on diaper area because child might inhale talc.

- Cloth diapers should be washed commercially, or presoaked in mild vinegar water before washing, to remove ammonia.

What You Can Do As a Parent

- Follow Caregiver recommendations.

Child May Return to School or Child Care . . .

Child need not be excluded from school or child care.

Possible Diagnosis: Candida Infection

What You Should Know

- Caused by a yeast infection within the intestines.

- Appears as a fiery red rash.

- Can be spread from child to child by an adult who does not wash hands thoroughly.

- Treated with prescription medication.

- Infection can also be present in mouth.

- Also see *Thrush* under *Mouth/Lip Eruptions* in this chart. (Both are caused by same organism.)

What You Can Do As a Caregiver

- Change diapers often; wear disposable gloves.

- Wash diaper area with soap and warm water; allow to dry completely.

- Do not use baby powder on diaper area because child might inhale talc.

- Wash hands thoroughly after removing gloves.

What You Can Do As a Parent

- Follow Caregiver recommendations.

- Call child's health care provider for prescription ointment and discuss treatment with oral medication.

Child May Return to School or Child Care . . .

when medication is started.

Diarrhea

What You Should Know

- Defined as several loose or watery stools.

- Caused primarily by viruses.

- Can also be caused by bacterial infections, antibiotics, and certain foods.

- May resolve without treatment within a few days if noninfectious.

- If mild diarrhea does not resolve within a few days, child should be seen by health care provider for stool culture to determine if diarrhea is infectious.

What You Can Do As a Caregiver

- See the section on *Diarrhea* in this chapter, and *Preventing Infection in a Child Care Setting* in Chapter 15.

What You Can Do as a Parent

- Follow Caregiver recommendations.

Child May Return to School or Child Care . . .

Child need not be excluded from school or child care if diarrhea can be contained in diaper or by normal toileting practices.

Possible Diagnosis: Infectious Diarrhea

What You Should Know

- An intestinal infection caused by bacteria such as *Salmonella* and *Shigella* species, a parasite such as *Giardia,* or a virus.

- Varies from mild to severe.

- Signs and symptoms:
  - Diarrhea containing blood or mucus
  - Stomach or abdominal cramping and gas
  - Foul-smelling stools
  - Fever
  - Weight loss

- Acquired by ingestion of contaminated water or food.

- Highly contagious.

- Diagnosed by stool culture(s).

- Treated with prescription medication.

- Infection should be reported to the local Department of Public Health by the child's health care provider.

What You Can Do As a Caregiver

- Wear disposable gloves for diapering or helping with toileting to reduce chances of spreading infection. Wash hands thoroughly after removing gloves.

- Encourage child to drink extra amounts of clear fluids.

- Do not allow child to share drinking glasses or eating utensils with others.

- Discuss treatment of all family members with health care provider.

- See the section on *Diarrhea* in this chapter, and *Preventing Infection in a Child Care Setting* in Chapter 15.

What You Can Do As a Parent

- Follow Caregiver recommendations.

- Contact child's health care provider.

Child May Return to School or Child Care . . .

if *Salmonella:* After treatment with antibiotics, and after 3 negative results on stool cultures. If *Shigella:* After treatment with antibiotics, after severe diarrhea is under control, and child is able to contain diarrhea with normal toileting practices. If *Giardia:* After treatment with prescription medication, after severe diarrhea is under control, and child is able to contain diarrhea with normal toileting practices. In all cases: Check with your health care consultant about your center's policy concerning a child's return after treatment for infectious diarrhea.

Common Childhood Illness Quick Reference

Diarrhea *(continued)*

Possible Diagnosis: Hepatitis A

What You Should Know

- An infection of the liver caused by a virus found in the intestines, and spread through the stool; not necessarily diarrhea.

- Spreads from person to person when hands contaminated with microscopic particles of stool touch food or eating utensils.

- Mild flu-like symptoms that develop 2 to 8 weeks after exposure.

- Contagious for 2 weeks before symptoms develop.

- Illness more serious in adults than in children.

- Should be reported to the local Department of Public Health by the health care provider

- No specific treatment.

What You Can Do As a Caregiver

- Also see *Infectious Diarrhea* above.

- Contact your health care provider if you are exposed to the Hepatitis A virus.

What You Can Do As a Parent

- Follow Caregiver recommendations.

- Contact the child's health care provider if any family member is exposed to the Hepatitis A virus.

Child May Return to School or Child Care . . .

child should remain at home while ill and may return when symptoms are no longer present and temperature is normal for 24 hours. Check with your health care consultant concerning a child's return following Hepatitis A infection.

Ear Pain

Possible Diagnosis: Otitis Media (Middle Ear Infection)

What You Should Know

- Can be painful.

- Often follows a cold that causes mucous blockage of the tube that connects throat and middle ear (eustachian tube), preventing drainage and allowing bacteria to cause infection.

- Signs and symptoms:
  - Repeated pulling of ear(s)
  - Cries of pain and general irritability
  - Fever
  - Fluid draining from ear(s)

- Treated with antibiotics.

- Not contagious.

- Some children have ear tubes inserted through the ear drum to allow fluid and pus to drain out through the ear canal. Special precautions must be taken to avoid getting water into ears during shampooing and swimming.

- Also see *Foreign Objects* in Chapter 7.

What You Can Do As a Caregiver

- Take temperature and treat as necessary with acetaminophen. Notify parent.

- Hold child in upright position to decrease pressure in ear and lessen pain.

- Do not allow child to drink from bottle while lying on the back, because this can encourage fluids containing mouth bacteria to enter eustachian tube and travel to middle ear.

- Never insert anything, including cotton swabs, into a child's ear.

- Watch for hearing loss or speech problem in child with recurring ear infections.

What You Can Do As a Parent

- Follow Caregiver recommendations.

- Call child's health care provider.

Child May Return to School or Child Care . . .

when child feels better and temperature is normal.

Common Childhood Illness Quick Reference

Eye Irritation/Pain

Possible Diagnosis: Conjunctivitis (Pink Eye)

What You Should Know

- Infection of the lining of the eye, often accompanying a cold.
- Signs and symptoms:
  - Red, irritated, or painful eye(s)
  - Yellow or watery drainage
  - Eyelids temporarily stuck together from encrusted discharge when child awakens from sleep
- Easily spread by touching infected secretions and then touching own eye area.
- Watery drainage is most likely viral conjunctivitis; resolves without treatment.
- Pus or yellow drainage is most likely bacterial conjunctivitis; must be treated with an antibiotic.

What You Can Do As a Caregiver

- Wear disposable gloves. Clean drainage from child's eye(s) with clean tissue or gauze pad and warm water, as needed. Wipe each eye outward from inner corner.
- Discourage touching eye(s).
- Wash hands thoroughly and encourage child to do the same.
- Notify parent if eye has pus or yellow drainage.
- See *Preventing Infection in a Child Care Setting* in Chapter 15.

What You Can Do As a Parent

- Follow Caregiver recommendations.
- Call child's health care provider.
- Wear disposable gloves. Apply ointment if prescribed: have child look upward; apply ointment to clean, cotton-tip applicator to avoid contaminating ointment tube; apply ointment on applicator to inside of lower eyelid.

Child May Return to School or Child Care . . .

when child is comfortable and eye discharge contains no pus, or after 24 hours of antibiotic treatment.

Possible Diagnosis: Sty

What You Should Know

- Infection of a sweat gland on the eye lid, usually near eye lashes.
- Appears as a painful red pimple.

What You Can Do As a Caregiver

- Wear disposable gloves.
- Apply warm wash cloth to eye for 5 to 10 minutes several times per day.
- Encourage child not to touch eyes.
- Wash hands thoroughly and encourage child to do the same.

What You Can Do As a Parent

- Follow Caregiver recommendations.
- Call child's health care provider if no improvement.

Child May Return to School or Child Care . . .

when child feels better.

Common Childhood Illness Quick Reference

Fever

Possible Diagnosis: Viral or Bacterial Infection

What You Should Know

- A child with a fever should not be in a child care setting.

What You Can Do As a Caregiver

- See the section on *Fever* in this chapter.

What You Can Do As a Parent

- See the section on *Fever* in this chapter.

Child May Return to School or Child Care . . .

when temperature is normal for 24 hours.

Headache

What You Should Know

- Most are minor and are caused by overexertion or stress.
- Might signal beginning of illness.
- Might signal problem with vision.

What You Can Do As a Caregiver

- Have child rest in a quiet, darkened area.
- Give acetaminophen as needed. Know your center's policy about use of acetaminophen. Report recurring headaches to parent.

What You Can Do As a Parent

- Have child rest in a quiet, darkened area.
- Give acetaminophen as needed. Call child's health care provider for recurrent headaches.

Child May Return to School or Child Care . . .

when child feels better.

Itching Scalp

Possible Diagnosis: Pediculosis Capitas (Head Lice) ▶ Figure 16-2

What You Should Know

- Infestation by a tiny parasitic insect on the scalp and hair.

- Signs and symptoms:

  - Persistent itching on scalp

  - Tiny red bites on scalp and on hairline

- Diagnosed by finding tiny yellow/white eggs, called nits, firmly attached to shaft of hair; adult lice are harder to find.

- Nits found all along hair shaft and all over head, but especially at crown, nape of neck, and behind ears.

- Most easily seen and removed when hair is partially or completely dry.

- Highly contagious.

- Transferred from person to person by crawling lice or sharing personal items such as hats, combs, and brushes.

- Not caused by uncleanliness.

- Lice cannot jump or fly.

- Not carried by cats or dogs.

- Requires thorough treatment of all family members who have head lice at the same time.

- Lice-killing shampoos are pesticides; use cautiously.

- Also see *Ringworm* under *Skin Eruptions and Rashes*.

What You Can Do As a Caregiver

- Notify child's parent.

- Notify all parents of a case of lice, but maintain confidentiality.

- Machine wash all washable items in hot water, including bed linens, blankets, towels, clothing, jackets, and hats.

- Use hot setting on dryer.

- Place pillows and stuffed animals in dryer on hot setting for 30 minutes.

- Place items that cannot be washed or dried in a closed plastic bag for 2 weeks.

- Vacuum upholstered furniture, mattresses, rugs, car seats, and stuffed toys.

- Do not use lice sprays.

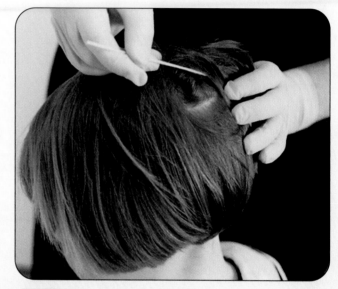

Figure 16-2 Checking for head lice.

What You Can Do As a Parent

- Follow Caregiver recommendations.

- Treat with lice-killing shampoo as recommended by child's health care provider. Follow package directions and wear disposable gloves when applying shampoo.

- Apply shampoo at the sink, never in the bathtub, to minimize skin exposed to pesticide.

- Safest if a pregnant or nursing mother does not apply shampoo, even if wearing gloves.

- Do not use lice-killing shampoo if cut or other open wound is present on scalp.

- Do not use lice-killing shampoo on infants.

- Treat all family members who have head lice at the same time.

- Remove all nits with small metal nit comb available in most pharmacies, or with fingernails.

- Check all family members' heads daily for 10 days.

- May have to repeat full treatment in 1 week.

- Scrub hair brushes, combs, and hair accessories, and then soak them in very hot water for 10 minutes.

Child May Return to School or Child Care . . .

after treatment with lice-killing shampoo and thorough nit removal. Know your center's or school's policy concerning a child's return after lice infestation.

Common Childhood Illness Quick Reference

Mouth/Lip Eruptions

Possible Diagnosis: Cold Sores (Herpes Simplex Virus) ▶ Figure 16-3

What You Should Know

- A viral disease that causes recurrent infections throughout life.
- Signs and symptoms:
  - Cluster of water blisters on lip
- Can be painful.
- Blisters break, weep, and scab over in several days.
- In children, the rash occurs almost exclusively on the face as a cold sore or fever blister.
- Child is contagious until all blisters have scabbed.
- Virus is spread by direct contact with the sore or by secretions from the sore.
- Infection recurs periodically.
- An adult or child who has an open herpes simplex sore on the mouth or other body area that cannot be completely covered should not be in a child care setting.
- No cure available.

What You Can Do As a Caregiver

- Keep area clean and dry.
- Do not touch an open cold sore.
- Wash hands thoroughly.

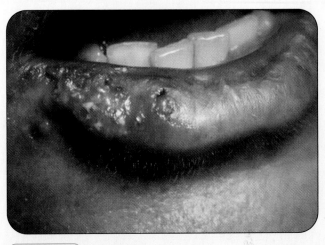

Figure 16-3 Cold sores.

What You Can Do As a Parent

- Follow Caregiver recommendations.

Child May Return to School or Child Care . . .

when an open sore has completely scabbed over, or can be completely covered.

Mouth/Lip Eruptions *(continued)*

Possible Diagnosis: Hand, Foot, and Mouth Syndrome

What You Should Know

- Mild viral infection.

- Usually occurs in children between 6 months and 4 years of age.

- Transmitted from person to person through saliva and stool.

- Incubation period is 3 to 6 days.

- Signs and symptoms:

  - Fever, sometimes as high as 104°F, lasting 3 to 4 days

  - Headache about 2 days before mouth sores develop

  - Ulcer-like sores in mouth, in throat, and on tongue, making eating and drinking difficult

  - Red spots that become blisters on palms and soles

  - Rash in the groin and on buttocks that seldom blister

- Child does not necessarily have spots or blisters in all locations.

- Illness resolves on its own in about 1 week.

- Typically seen in summer and fall.

- Dehydration can occur in a young child who refuses to drink because of mouth sores.

What You Can Do As a Caregiver

- Take child's temperature, and contact parent to pick up child.

- Separate child from group.

What You Can Do As a Parent

- Give acetaminophen for fever over 101°F, and for pain in mouth.

- Use over-the-counter products to numb mouth sores.

- Rinse mouth with lukewarm water after eating.

- Boil silverware or use disposable utensils to avoid transmitting disease.

- Boil bottle nipples for 20 minutes.

- Encourage fluids as tolerated, including popsicles; milk is often soothing.

- Offer soft foods, including ice cream, sherbet, gelatin, pudding, soft breads, noodles, and rice.

- Avoid citrus fruits, salty or spicy foods, carbonated beverages, crunchy cereals, and other foods requiring chewing.

- Do not break blisters on hands and feet; they heal better if not broken.

Child May Return to School or Child Care . . .

when mouth sores and blisters are healed, approximately 1 week.

Possible Diagnosis: Thrush

What You Should Know

- A yeast infection in the mouth.

- Appears as white patches on the mucous membranes of the mouth and on the tongue.

- Easily spreads from one infant to another.

- Seldom occurs in infants over 6 months of age.

- Must be treated with antifungal medication.

- Also see *Candida Infection* under *Diaper Rash*.

What You Can Do As a Caregiver

- Wear disposable gloves when handling items the child has mouthed to reduce the chance of infection spreading to others.

- Wash hands thoroughly after removing gloves.

- Carefully wash all items that might reinfect child, such as nipples, pacifier, and mouthed toys.

- Do not allow babies to share mouthed toys, pacifiers, or bottles.

What You Can Do As a Parent

- Follow Caregiver recommendations.

Child May Return to School or Child Care . . .

when treatment has started.

Common Childhood Illness Quick Reference

Runny Nose

Possible Diagnosis: Cold

See the section on *Colds* in this chapter.

Skin Eruptions and Rashes

Possible Diagnosis: Chicken Pox ▶ Figure 16-4

What You Should Know

- A common viral illness lasting approximately 1 week.

- Incubation period is 10 to 21 days.

- Contagious from 1 to 2 days before rash appears until all blisters have scabbed over (about 1 week).

- Rash of red bumps appears primarily on face and trunk as fluid-filled bubbles that break, weep, and scab.

- Rash can also appear on arms, legs, or any mucous membrane surface, such as inside the mouth, throat, eyes, and vagina.

- Other signs and symptoms:

  - Fever

  - Itching

- Is spread by nose or throat secretions containing chicken pox virus, or by touching rash.

- Dry scabs are not contagious.

- One bout provides immunity.

- Vaccine available.

What You Can Do As a Caregiver

- Wear disposable gloves and wash hands thoroughly after removing gloves.

- Take temperature and treat for fever as necessary. Know your center's policy concerning the use of acetaminophen.

- Notify parent.

- See the section on *Fever* in this chapter.

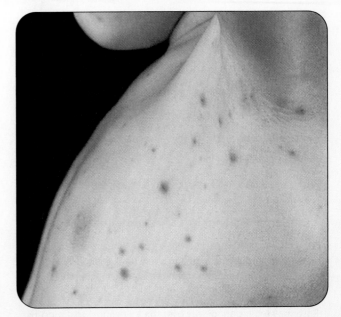

Figure 16-4 Chicken Pox.

What You Can Do As a Parent

- Encourage child to drink clear fluids.

- Bathe child in warm water with $^1/_2$ cup baking soda or 1 to 2 cups colloidal oatmeal to relieve itching.

- Apply calamine lotion to relieve itching; avoid eyes.

- Call child's health care provider, who might recommend a medicine for itching.

- Trim child's fingernails or put mittens on infant to prevent scratching, which can infect open lesions and lead to scarring.

- Avoid giving aspirin.

- Notify child's health care provider if child is unusually uncomfortable, cannot drink, has persistent high fever, severe headache, or is disoriented.

- Watch for chicken pox to develop in other family members or playmates for 3 weeks.

Child May Return to School or Child Care . . .

when all blisters have scabbed over, approximately 7 days.

Common Childhood Illness Quick Reference

Skin Eruptions and Rashes (continued)

Possible Diagnosis: Fifth Disease ▶ Figure 16-5

What You Should Know

- Mild viral illness, harmless for most children.

- Incubation period is 4 to 14 days.

- Contagious several days before appearance of rash.

- Signs and symptoms:

  - Bright red rash on cheeks, giving face a "slapped cheek" appearance

  - Lacy red rash on arms, legs, and trunk; usually gone in 10 days

- Other symptoms, which pass in a few days, include: low-grade fever, fatigue, headache, sore throat, stomach ache, chills, and decreased appetite.

- Rash may recur periodically over the following 3 to 4 months, usually due to sunlight, warm baths, or emotional upset; child will not be contagious.

- Spreads through contact with throat and mouth secretions.

- Can be serious for children with some chronic illnesses such as sickle cell anemia and thalessemia, or with suppressed immune systems, such as leukemia and AIDS patients.

- May present risk to fetus.

- No vaccine available.

- One bout of infection is believed to provide lifelong immunity.

What You Can Do As a Caregiver

- Wear disposable gloves and wash hands thoroughly after removing gloves.

- Take temperature and treat for fever as necessary. Know your center's policy concerning the use of acetaminophen.

- Notify all parents because of possible health risks to unborn babies and to children with serious illnesses. A pregnant woman who is exposed to fifth disease should consult her health care provider.

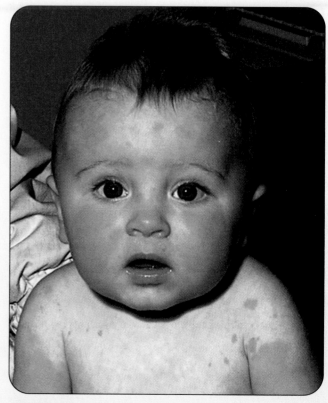

Figure 16-5 Fifth disease.

What You Can Do As a Parent

- Give acetaminophen for fever and headache.

- Contact child's health care provider.

Child May Return to School or Child Care . . .

Child need not be excluded from school or child care if temperature is normal and child feels well.

Common Childhood Illness Quick Reference

Skin Eruptions and Rashes *(continued)*

Possible Diagnosis: Heat Rash (Prickly Heat)

What You Should Know

- Experienced mostly by infants and young children.

- Characterized by tiny pink bumps in areas that tend to be moist.

- Commonly seen in skin folds of neck and on upper chest, arms, legs, and diaper area.

- Occurs during hot and humid weather.

- Clears up in a few days.

What You Can Do As a Caregiver

- Pay special attention to skin folds that stay wet with perspiration, urine, or drool.

- Apply calamine lotion to reddest areas.

- Leave areas open to air, without clothing.

- Allow fan to blow gently on child when sleeping.

- Do not apply skin ointments.

- Use powder in sparse amounts by pouring a small amount into your hand, away from child's face, and applying to skin so powder is barely visible. Be aware that use of powder is generally not recommended for children because of risk of inhalation of talc.

What You Can Do As a Parent

- Follow Caregiver recommendations.

- Bathe child without soap.

- Allow skin to air dry.

Child May Return to School or Child Care . . .

Child need not be excluded from school or child care.

Possible Diagnosis: Impetigo ▶ Figure 16-6

What You Should Know

- A streptococcal or staphylococcal bacterial skin infection that can develop after an insect bite, cut, or other break in the skin.

- Commonly seen on the face but can develop in any skin injury such as insect bite or cut.

- Signs and symptoms:

  - Red, oozing rash covered by fine, honey-colored scab

  - Pain and itching

- Can spread to other parts of child's body if child scratches.

- Can spread to others in close contact by direct touching or touching a surface contaminated with secretions.

- Requires topical antibiotic ointment treatment.

- Infection more worrisome in infants than in older children.

What You Can Do As a Caregiver

- Notify parent.

- Discourage scratching.

- Trim fingernails.

- Do not permit sharing of towels or face cloths.

- Wear disposable gloves while caring for infected skin to reduce chance of infection spreading to you and others.

- Wash hands thoroughly after removing gloves.

- Observe rash and note any improvement or worsening.

What You Can Do As a Parent

- Follow Caregiver recommendations.

- Call child's health care provider for antibiotic ointment recommendation.

- Remove scab by soaking before applying antibiotic ointment.

Child May Return to School or Child Care . . .

24 hours after treatment is started.

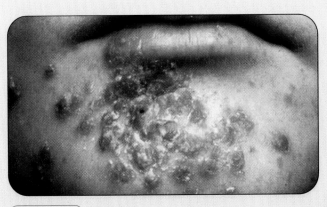

Figure 16-6 Impetigo.

Common Childhood Illness Quick Reference

Skin Eruptions and Rashes *(continued)*

Possible Diagnosis: Ringworm ▼ Figure 16-7

What You Should Know

- A minor infection that is mildly contagious.

- A superficial fungal infection of the skin, affecting young children primarily on the scalp and trunk.

- Scalp infection causes temporary bald patches, 1/2" to 2" in diameter.

- On trunk, infection causes round or oval, red, scaly patches that spread outward and heal in the center, resembling a doughnut.

- Infection cannot penetrate skin but sits on the surface.

- Spreads from person to person by direct contact with ringworm lesion.

- Treated with antifungal topical cream that must be used for several weeks after rash disappears.

- No longer contagious 48 hours after treatment.

What You Can Do As a Caregiver

- Notify parent at end of day.

- Wash hands thoroughly and encourage child to do the same.

What You Can Do As a Parent

- Wear disposable gloves when applying over-the-counter antifungal cream or ointment.

- Continue to use cream or ointment for several weeks after rash disappears.

- Wash hands thoroughly after removing gloves.

Child May Return to School or Child Care ...

immediately after treatment is started.

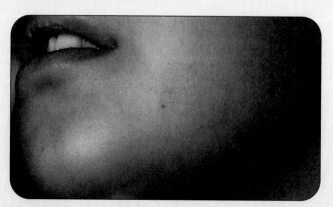

Figure 16-7 Ringworm.

Possible Diagnosis: Roseola ▼ Figure 16-8

What You Should Know

- A viral illness occurring in young children primarily under 2 years of age.

- Incubation period is 5 to 15 days.

- Mildly contagious.

- Characterized by a persistent high fever (103°F or higher) for 3 to 4 days without other symptoms.

- Fever drops suddenly about day 4, and generalized red rash appears over the entire body.

- Rash is gone in about 24 hours.

- One bout provides immunity.

What You Can Do As a Caregiver

- Take temperature and treat for fever as necessary. Know your center's policy concerning the use of acetaminophen.

- Notify parent.

- Encourage the child to drink clear fluids.

What You Can Do As a Parent

- Call child's health care provider.

- See the section on *Fever* in this chapter.

Child May Return to School or Child Care ...

when child feels better and temperature is normal for 24 hours.

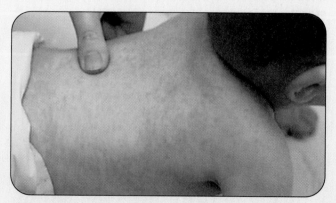

Figure 16-8 Roseola.

Common Childhood Illness Quick Reference

Skin Eruptions and Rashes *(continued)*

Possible Diagnosis: Scabies

What You Should Know

- A parasitic infection caused by mites that burrow under the superficial layer of skin.

- Incubation period is up to 30 days.

- Causes intense itching.

- Often seen in moist areas of the body, such as groin, buttocks, webbed spaces of fingers and toes, and underarms.

- Burrows first appear as fine, gray lines under the skin; area of infection enlarges as adult mites burrow and lay eggs under the skin.

- Diagnosed by skin scraping in which mite or egg is seen.

- Transferred by close body contact and shared clothing.

- Mites cannot jump or fly.

- Child must be treated at home with prescription mite-killing cream or lotion.

- Itching might last 2 to 4 weeks after treatment.

What You Can Do As a Caregiver

- Notify child's parent.

- Notify all other parents of a case of scabies, but maintain confidentiality.

- Machine wash all washable items in hot water, including bed linens, blankets, towels, clothing, jackets, and hats.

- Use hot setting on dryer.

- Place pillows and stuffed animals in a dryer on hot setting for 30 minutes.

- Leave items that cannot be washed or dried in a closed plastic bag for 4 days.

- Vacuum upholstered furniture, rugs, and car seats.

- Do not use mite sprays.

- Discourage child from scratching.

What You Can Do As a Parent

- Follow Caregiver recommendations.

- Wear disposable gloves when applying the mite-killing lotion. Follow package directions.

- Wash hands thoroughly after removing gloves.

- Bathe child 8 to 10 hours later to wash off lotion.

- Check with child's health care provider about repeating full treatment in 1 week.

- Do not use mite-killing lotion on infants.

- Treat all infected family members at the same time.

Child May Return to School or Child Care . . .

1 day after treatment is applied.

Common Childhood Illness Quick Reference

Skin Eruptions and Rashes *(continued)*

Possible Diagnosis: Scarlet Fever (Scarlatina)

▶ Figure 16-9

What You Should Know

- A streptococcal bacterial infection that causes a generalized illness.

- More serious than simple "strep" throat.

- Incubation period is 2 to 5 days.

- Contagious—spreads from person to person by direct contact and by inhaling tiny droplets of infected secretions from nose.

- Signs and symptoms:

  - Rash appears primarily on trunk and is most intense at underarms, on groin, behind knees, and on inner thighs

  - Rash resembles a sunburn covered with tiny "goosebumps"

  - Rash starts on chest and spreads downward

  - Painful sore throat

  - High fever

  - Tongue has white coating that changes to strawberry color after 4 to 5 days

  - Nausea and vomiting

  - Skin peels after 1 week

- Treated with an antibiotic.

- If untreated the child may be at risk for developing rheumatic fever.

What You Can Do As a Caregiver

- Take temperature and treat for fever as necessary. Know your center's policy concerning the use of acetaminophen.

- Give child throat lozenges to suck.

- Encourage child to drink clear fluids.

- Wash hands thoroughly after caring for child to reduce chance of spreading infection to yourself and others.

- Notify parent.

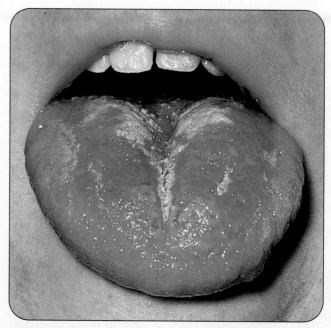

Figure 16-9 Scarlet fever.

What You Can Do As a Parent

- Wash hands thoroughly after caring for child.

- Call child's health care provider.

Child May Return to School or Child Care . . .

24 hours after antibiotic treatment has started, when temperature is normal for 24 hours, and when child feels well.

Common Childhood Illness Quick Reference

Sore Throat

Possible Diagnosis: Viral Sore Throat

What You Should Know

- Contagious.
- Will get better without treatment.
- More than 90% of sore throats are viral.

What You Can Do As a Caregiver

- Take temperature and treat for fever as necessary. Know your center's policy concerning the use of acetaminophen.
- Wash hands thoroughly after caring for child.
- Do not allow child to share mouthed toys, pacifiers, bottles, cups, or eating utensils.

What You Can Do As a Parent

- Follow Caregiver recommendations.
- Call child's health care provider for throat culture if symptoms persist for more than 2 to 3 days.

Child May Return to School or Child Care . . .

when temperature is normal.

Possible Diagnosis: "Strep" Throat

What You Should Know

- A streptococcal bacterial infection.
- Occurs much less often than a viral throat infection but is more serious.
- Abrupt onset.
- Highly contagious—spreads from person to person by direct contact and by inhaling tiny droplets of infected secretions from nose.
- Incubation period of 2 to 5 days.
- Child is infectious only after symptoms appear and remains infectious until antibiotics have been taken for at least 24 hours.
- Signs and symptoms:
  - Persistent, painful sore throat, especially when swallowing
  - White patches on throat and tonsils
  - Persistent fever
  - Swollen glands
  - Headache
  - Nausea and vomiting
- Can be serious, if untreated, with possible later damage to heart and kidneys.
- Requires throat culture to diagnose.
- Treated with antibiotic.
- Also see *Scarlet Fever* under *Skin Eruptions and Rashes*.

What You Can Do As a Caregiver

- Take temperature and treat for fever as necessary. Know your center's policy concerning the use of acetaminophen.
- Wash hands thoroughly after caring for child.
- Do not allow child to share mouthed toys, pacifiers, bottles, cups, or eating utensils.

What You Can Do As a Parent

- Follow Caregiver recommendations.
- Complete entire course of antibiotic treatment to prevent relapse, even if child appears to recover quickly.

Child May Return to School or Child Care . . .

after 24 hours of antibiotic treatment and when temperature is normal.

Common Childhood Illness Quick Reference

Tooth Pain

Possible Diagnosis: Bottlemouth ▸ Figure 16-10

What You Should Know

• Special form of tooth decay in very young children.

• Caused by lengthy exposure to milk or other liquids containing sugar at naptime and bedtime.

• Most common in upper front teeth.

• Treatment often requires oral surgery with general anesthesia.

What You Can Do As a Caregiver

• Do not give child a bottle of milk or juice (or any fluid containing sugar) at nap or bedtime. Give only water, or eliminate sleep time bottle.

What You Can Do As a Parent

• Follow Caregiver recommendations.

Child May Return to School or Child Care . . .

Child need not be excluded from school or child care.

Possible Diagnosis: Cavities

What You Should Know

• Caused by sticky foods that leave sugar coating on teeth.

• Affects children age 3 and older.

What You Can Do As a Caregiver

• Avoid giving child sticky foods that cling to teeth and cause decay, such as raisins, gummy fruit-flavored treats, caramel candy, and licorice.

• Encourage child to eat popcorn, pretzels, raw vegetables, fresh fruit, and yogurt.

• Encourage child to brush teeth after snacks and meals. Use toothpaste with fluoride when child is old enough to spit it out instead of swallowing it.

What You Can Do As a Parent

• Follow Caregiver recommendations.

Child May Return to School or Child Care . . .

Child need not be excluded from school or child care.

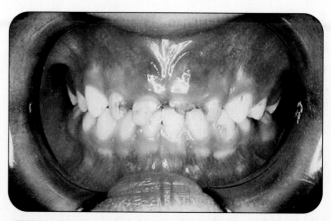

Figure 16-10 Bottlemouth.

Possible Diagnosis: Teething

What You Should Know

• Gum pain caused by newly erupting teeth.

• Can cause exaggerated crankiness.

• Can be very painful and cause sleepless nights.

• Can be accompanied by low-grade fever (<102°F).

What You Can Do As a Caregiver

• Provide teething toys for the child to chew.

• Do not rub child's gum with your finger.

• Use over-the-counter topical teething products. Know your center's policy about the use of these products.

• Wear disposable gloves.

• Wash hands thoroughly after removing gloves.

What You Can Do As a Parent

• Follow Caregiver recommendations.

• Contact child's health care provider if fever exceeds 102°F because the child might also have an infection.

Child May Return to School or Child Care . . .

Child need not be excluded from school or child care if temperature is normal.

Common Childhood Illness Quick Reference

Urination, Painful

Possible Diagnosis: Urinary Tract Infection

What You Should Know

- Infection usually caused by bacteria.
- Signs and symptoms:
  - Strong burning sensation on urination
  - Feelings of frequent and urgent need to urinate
  - Urinating in small amounts
- More common in girls than boys because of short urethra and close proximity to anus.

What You Can Do As a Caregiver

- Notify child's parent.
- Encourage child to drink fluids.
- Teach girls to wipe only from front to back after toileting.

What You Can Do As a Parent

- Follow Caregiver recommendations.
- Call child's health care provider promptly.
- Child needs to give urine specimen and be treated with antibiotic.
- Avoid using bubble baths because these products can irritate the urethra in boys and girls.

Child May Return to School or Child Care . . .

Child need not be excluded from school or child care.

Vomiting

Possible Diagnosis: Viral Gastrointestinal Infection

What You Should Know

- Many are contagious.
- Less often caused by food poisoning or emotional upset.
- Also see the section on *Vomiting* in this chapter.

What You Can Do As a Caregiver

- Wear disposable gloves when handling vomit.
- Wash hands thoroughly after removing gloves.
- Remove child from the group.
- Notify parent.
- Give no food or fluid until 1 hour after vomiting has stopped.

What You Can Do As a Parent

- See the section on *Vomiting* in this chapter.

Child May Return to School or Child Care . . .

the following day if child feels better and temperature is normal.

Learning Activities

Common Childhood Illnesses

Directions: Circle Yes if you agree with the statement, and circle No if you disagree.

Yes   No   **1.** Fifth disease can present a risk to an unborn baby.

Yes   No   **2.** Antibiotics can cause diarrhea.

Yes   No   **3.** Lice can jump and fly from person to person.

Yes   No   **4.** Diarrhea is less worrisome in infants than older children.

Yes   No   **5.** A fever helps in fighting an illness.

Yes   No   **6.** Sponge bathing a child with tepid water helps to reduce a fever.

Yes   No   **7.** Vomiting can cause dehydration.

Yes   No   **8.** Apple juice is helpful in stopping diarrhea.

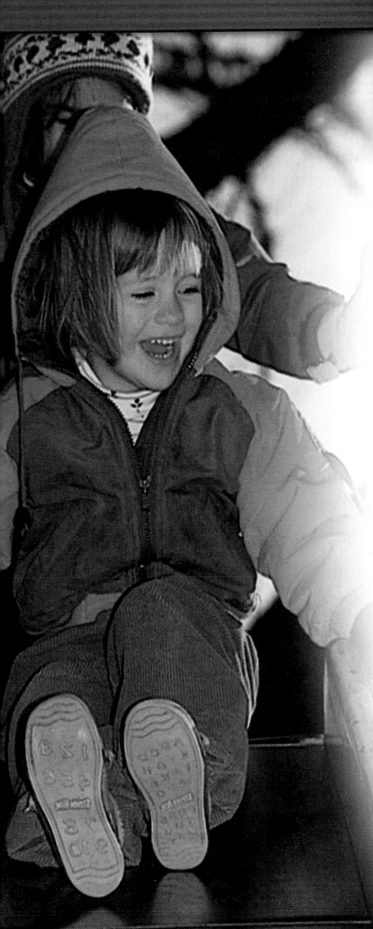

Chapter 17

Preventing Childhood Injury

Young children will naturally learn about their environment by exploring, particularly with their senses of taste and touch. Because they cannot make judgments about their own health and safety, this puts them at risk for injuries such as burns, falls, choking, drowning, and poisoning.

A child care provider's understanding of a child's growth and development is invaluable in creating a hazard-free environment with safe, age-appropriate items. It is essential to identify and remove all potential dangers. Safety is an even greater challenge in family child care settings and homes, because children are likely to be of different ages and at different developmental stages. Creative spacing of play areas and thoughtful storage of toys may be required.

As children grow, the hazards they face change because of their advancing capabilities. Remember that a mobile child's possibilities for adventure—both horizontal and vertical—are endless.

This chapter has general information on preventing childhood injury. Specific information on preventing burn injuries and fires is in Chapter 6, and information on preventing poisonings is in Chapter 9.

Indoor Safety

Spend some time in each room of the child care center or home examining it for safety hazards that might injure a child.

Bathroom

- Keep the toilet lid down. Do not use continuous blue or bleach-containing bowl cleaners.
- Keep the bathroom door closed to keep very young children out.
- Use a rubber mat or nonskid decals in the bathtub and shower stall.
- Pad the bath tub faucet to prevent injury.
- Set the temperature of the water heater to 120°F. See *Preventing Burn Injuries* in Chapter 6.
- Keep electrical appliances used in the bathroom, such as blow dryers, away from water.
- Do not store medicines or chemicals in the bathroom.

Common Injuries Related to Child's Developmental Level

Developmental Characteristics	Potential Injuries
Infant—Age 0 to 1 year	
Increasing mobility	Burns
Uses mouth to explore objects	Choking
Reaches for and pulls objects	Drowning
Unaware of dangers	Falls
Cannot understand "no"	
Toddler—Age 1 to 2½ years	
Masters walking, running, climbing	Burns
Explores almost everything with mouth	Choking
Begins to imitate behaviors	Drowning
Investigates everything within reach	Falls
Curious about all never-before-seen items	Pedestrian injuries
Unaware of most dangers	Poisoning
Impulsive	Suffocation
Preschooler—Age 2½ to 5 years	
Mobility leads to increased independence	Burns
	Choking
Learns to ride tricycle	Drowning
Unaware of many dangers	Falls
Might favor real, rather than toy, tools, gadgets, appliances	Pedestrian injuries
Fascinated with fire	Poisoning
Imitates adult behavior	
School-aged—Age 5 years and up	
Needs to be independent	Bicycle injuries
Needs to be like peers	Burns
Needs to be with peers	Falls
Needs increased physical activity	Pedestrian injuries
Dangers do not always seem real	
Increased independence can mean less supervision	Firearm injuries

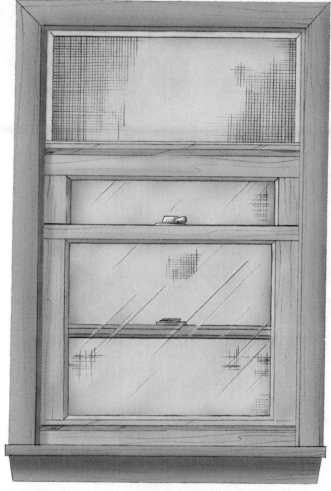

Figure 17-1) Open double hung windows from the top.

Sleeping Area

- Crib: see *Infant Equipment Safety* in this chapter.
- Never leave a baby unattended on a changing table, even if the infant is strapped.
- Change clothes and diapers of active infants and toddlers on the floor rather than on a table.
- Do not place any furniture that a child might climb on under a bedroom window.
- Open double-hung windows from the top down to prevent a fall from the window. Some states and private agencies provide financial support for obtaining child-safety screens for windows ▲ **Figure 17-1**). Check with your local Public Health Department.
- Do not let a child sit on a windowsill.
- Use a bed side guard when a child first uses a bed.
- Use a bed side guard for a top bunk. Do not allow young children to play or sleep on the top bunk.

Garage, Basement, and Laundry Area

Children should be kept out of these areas if hazardous chemicals and equipment are stored without child safety in mind.

- Install a hook and eye latch above the child's reach on the entrance door to these areas.
- Keep chemicals in their original containers. Place them on high shelves or in a locked cabinet. Purchase corrosive chemicals such as drain cleaners in one-use packages.
- Avoid interruptions when using a poisonous product. If you must leave your work area, put the chemical safely away or carry it with you.
- Store ropes and cords out of the reach of children.
- Keep the washer and dryer doors closed.
- Lock a freezer or extra refrigerator.

Kitchen

- Cook on back burners to prevent children from touching hot elements or flame. See *Preventing Burn Injuries* in Chapter 6.
- Do not store household cleaning products next to foods. The differences between them might not be apparent to a young child.
- Keep products in their original, labeled containers. Do not reuse containers such as juice bottles or empty food containers.
- Use plastic latches or other safety latches on kitchen cupboards and drawers that contain dangerous items such as knives.
- Keep heavy objects and appliances with cords, such as blenders, food processors, or small TVs away from the edge of the countertop or table so that a young child cannot reach them.
- Do not allow a child to play at your feet while you are cooking.
- To prevent falls, wipe up spills immediately and limit the use of floor wax or polish.
- Position a high chair so that a child cannot reach the stove, countertop, or electric or phone cords. See *Infant Equipment Safety* in this chapter.
- Do not allow children to chew on styrofoam cups and food containers. Particles can be inhaled and cause respiratory irritation.

Living Area

- Check smoke detector batteries in the spring and fall when you change your clocks. See *Preventing Burn Injuries* in Chapter Six.
- Anchor tall and unsteady bookcases to the walls.
- Rearrange furniture if sharp corners on tables protrude into areas of heavy traffic.
- Do not leave dangerous items such as hot beverages or sharp scissors on a low table.
- Place decorative stickers at a child's eye level on sliding glass doors to prevent a child from colliding with the glass.

Stairs

- Be cautious when using expandable doorway gates at stairwells. If you use an accordion-type gate with large diamond-shaped openings, be sure the gate has a safety rail along the top to eliminate the V-shaped openings where children can entrap their heads. Safer gate models are tension gates made entirely of plastic or plastic mesh on a wooden frame, which snap closed in doorways. Use gates only for the doorway widths suggested by the manufacturer. Do not climb over a doorway gate yourself because children often mimic adults.
- Make stairs skid-proof with carpet or rubber mats. Place skid-proof padding under all small area rugs or hallway rugs.
- Repair or replace torn carpeting on the stairs to prevent tripping and falling.
- Check that handrails are secured to the wall.
- Keep the stairway area well lit and unblocked.
- Teach young children to descend stairs by crawling down backwards.

Inside or Outside the Building

- Test paint on the windows, the windowsills and the building exterior for lead content. Call your Department of Public Health to learn about the proper procedures. If it is necessary to remove the lead, children must not be present. See *Lead Poisoning in Children* in this chapter.
- Test your center or home for the presence of radon. Radon is a lung-cancer-causing radioactive gas that you cannot see, smell, or taste. It comes from the natural breakdown of uranium under the ground and it gets into buildings through cracks in the basement or other foundations. There are many ways to solve a radon problem in a building. Obtain a testing kit in your local hardware store or by contacting your state radon office. For more information, call the National Radon Hotline at 1-800-SOS-RADON.

Infant Equipment Safety

Young children are active, whether on the floor or in one of the many pieces of equipment designed to meet their needs and yours. Because they cannot evaluate possible hazards, they can be injured in what seems to be the safest of places.

Standards and guidelines for juvenile equipment have been improved over the years by the U.S. Consumer Product Safety Commission. Check older equipment before using it, to make certain that it conforms to current standards and guidelines.

Cribs

Current federal regulations require the following:

- Standard-size cribs must have mattresses that fit snugly. If two fingers can fit between the mattress and the crib, the mattress is too small ▼ **Figure 17-2**).

- Crib slats must be no more than $2^3/8''$ apart so that infants cannot slip through and become strangled or trapped. Do not use a crib with decorative openings in the end panels that could trap a head or limb. Do not use a crib with a broken or missing slat.

- Corner posts must not stick up above the front and back panels by more than $1/16''$ to prevent entanglement of clothing.

- There must be no rough edges or metal hardware inside the crib.

- Locks on the side rails must not be accessible to a child, who might release them.

Your responsibility checklist includes:

- Make sure that the metal mattress support hangers are secure on the headboard and footboard posts.

- Do not allow drapery or blind cords to hang near a crib. Do not string toys from rail to rail or across a crib. Both present a risk for strangulation.

- Use crib bumper pads, mobiles, and crib gyms only until the child can push up onto hands and knees; then remove them.

- When the child can pull up to stand, lower the crib mattress to the lowest position.

- Immediately remove and replace a cracked plastic teething rail.

- Never use plastic bags to cover mattresses or pillows.

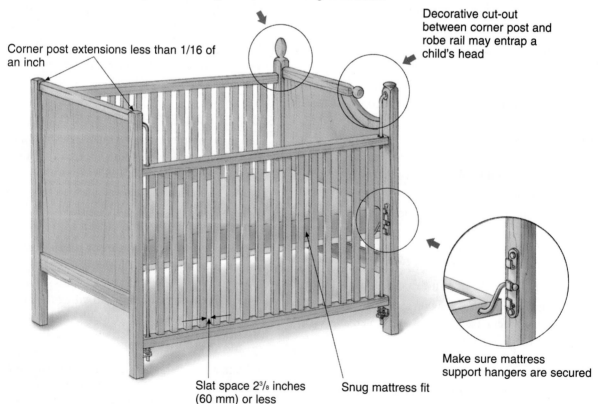

Corner post extensions greater than 1/16 of an inch (1 1/2 mm) may cause entanglement with clothing or necklace

Decorative cut-out between corner post and robe rail may entrap a child's head

Corner post extensions less than 1/16 of an inch

Slat space 2³/₈ inches (60 mm) or less

Snug mattress fit

Make sure mattress support hangers are secured

(**Figure 17-2**) Crib regulations help to keep infants safe.

- Do not put a pillow in the crib with an infant.

- Place only small soft toys in a crib; a child can stand on large ones, leading to a fall.

- Stop using the crib once the height of the top rails is less than three fourths of the child's height, usually when the child reaches about 35″.

- Place an infant on the side or back for sleep; this may help reduce the risk of a sudden infant death.

Lead Poisoning in Children

The toxic effects of lead on the human body have caused the United States government to name it the country's number one environmental threat to children. Unlike many environmental health problems, lead is often found right at home—in drinking water, household paint, house dust, and outdoor soil. Lead is especially damaging to children under age 6. The tragedy of lead poisoning is that there are no warning signs in the early stages. Often the poisoning is not diagnosed until there is some degree of irreparable brain damage causing developmental delays, behavioral problems, and intellectual impairment. There is recent evidence that lead is toxic at blood levels once thought safe. Lower IQ scores, slower development, attention problems, and kidney and stomach problems have been observed in children with very low levels of lead in their blood. Screening children for lead is generally done between 1 and 2 years of age, or earlier if the child's risk of exposure is high.

Infants and toddlers can come in contact with lead-contaminated dust and soil because they spend a lot of time on the floor or ground and often have their hands in their mouths. Most buildings constructed before 1960 have some lead paint inside or on the exterior, which ends up in the air or the soil as the paint ages. Even more serious are the higher doses of lead that young children receive when they eat tiny chips of old leaded paint. Lead dust can be found in high concentrations in building renovations where lead paint is disturbed, and on windows, windowsills, or on older porch floors where it is ground up by the friction of walking. Some older buildings also have lead water pipes and lead-soldered copper pipes that can leach lead into the water, especially into hot water. Some other sources of lead include lead-glazed pottery and some imported painted toys. To prevent children from ingesting lead, be sure to test water, paint, and soil levels and make the necessary corrections.

High Chairs

High chairs allow children to explore food and to feed themselves with a minimum of kitchen mess. However, adult supervision is necessary.

Your responsibility checklist includes:

- Never leave a child unattended in a high chair.

- Use a high chair with both a lap and a crotch strap. Always fasten the straps. From the first time the high chair is introduced, the child must understand that being safely secured is part of the eating process.

- If the high chair has a detachable tray, teach the child to raise the hands over the head while you attach the tray to prevent pinched fingers.

- Do not allow a child to climb into a high chair unassisted or to stand on the seat.

Playpens

Playpens can provide a safe play environment when there are tasks or other children that require your full attention.

Your responsibility checklist includes:

- Check that the weave of the mesh-netting sides is tiny enough so that small items cannot be pushed into the playpen by other children.

- Do not place large toys in a playpen. Children can stand on them and fall out.

- Do not hang toys with cords across the playpen because of the risk of strangulation.

- Remove the playpen once the child is able to climb over the side.

- Never leave the sides of a mesh playpen in the down position. Infants can suffocate by becoming trapped between the mesh and the plastic mattress.

- Measure the slats on an older wooden playpen. If the space between slats is larger than $2^{3}/_{8}″$, there is a risk that the child will become trapped between them.

Walkers and Stationary Exercisers

Walkers enable older infants to walk around before they have mastered this task on their own. In fact, it is surprising how fast an infant can propel a walker. Unfortunately, many injuries to infants have occurred as a result of the access to unsafe areas and items that a walker provides. In addition, walkers can easily tip over. Because of the unusually large number of walker-related injuries, their use is not recommended.

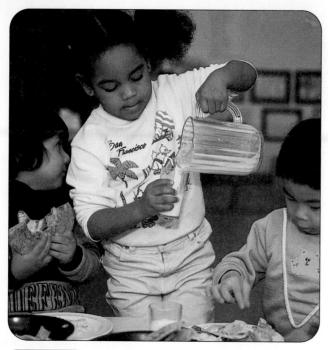

Figure 17-3 Make certain that children are only offered age-appropriate foods.

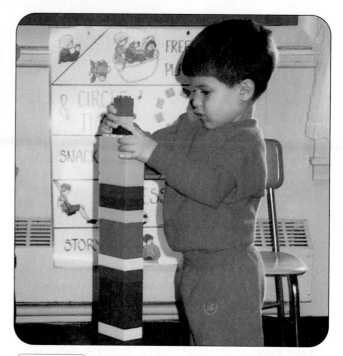

Figure 17-4 Make certain that a child has access to safe, age-appropriate toys.

Manufacturers also offer walker-like, stationary exercisers called saucers that spin, bounce, and rock. These look very much like walkers but eliminate the ability to move around. Although saucers are safer than walkers, some experts caution that both should be used for only short periods of time. Walkers and stationary exercisers place children in an upright position before their muscles are ready and puts undue stress on the back.

Choking Prevention

Choking is one of the leading causes of death to children and is most often experienced by children under 3 years of age (▲ **Figure 17-3**). Although children can choke on small household items, coins, and toy parts, food is the most common cause of choking. Read about emergency care for choking, or airway obstruction, in Chapter 3.

Safety rules to prevent choking include:

* Keep all small items away from young children.

* Teach children not to speak with food in the mouth. A laugh or sudden gasp can direct food into the airway.

* Make certain that children sit while eating.

* Cut up or break food into small pieces.

* Avoid giving the following foods to children under 1 year of age and give only with supervision to children between 1 and 3 years of age:

Apple peels	Marshmallows
Bony fish	Nuts
Chewing gum	Oranges
Corn kernels	Peanut butter
Grapes	Popcorn
Hard candy	Raisins
Hotdogs	Raw carrots
Ice	Raw celery

Toy Safety

Government regulations on newly manufactured toys reduce potential hazards and help to maintain high standards for American-made toys. These regulations, together with good faith compliance and testing by the industry, make toys for today's children safer than those of the generations before them. However, not all toy-related injuries can be prevented by government regulations and the toy industry.

Toy manufacturers label toys with age recommendations and, although they are sound recommendations, they are only a guide. Consider the developmental stages, the style of play, and interests of the children (▲ **Figure 17-4**). Do they play vigorously? Do they mouth toys?

Guidelines for preventing toy injuries include:

* Read labels. Look for the manufacturer's age recommendations. Allow young children to play only with toys or toy parts that are too large to become lodged in the throat.

- Check each toy carefully, making sure that no small part can be pulled off. Check for sharp points or edges, exposed wires, and torn seams.
- Choose toys that hold up well to repeated use.
- Discard plastic packaging immediately.
- Never repair toys for a young child who tends to throw toys or mouth them. Discard broken toys immediately.
- Sand wooden toys with rough edges.
- Be cautious in purchasing toys from foreign markets because some are painted with lead paint.
- Keep uninflated balloons and small balloon pieces out of the reach of children.
- Do not permit loud toys.
- Purchase only nontoxic art supplies.
- Teach children to put toys away. Toys left on the floor become a safety hazard.
- Store toys in plastic storage containers or in toy boxes with plastic lids and air holes or with spring-loaded hinges. Heavy, free-falling lids are responsible for many injuries.
- Store toys with small parts for older children separately from toys for younger children.
- Do not allow a child to dress up in a cape or scarf that touches the floor. The child's neck might be injured if someone steps on the material from behind.
- Make sure that batteries in toys are inaccessible to children.

For infants:

- Use only rattles and squeeze toys that are too large to become lodged in the throat.
- Do not hang toys with long cords or strings in or across a crib or playpen due to the risk of strangulation. Remove long ribbons or strings from stuffed animals. Also see the tips under *Cribs* in this chapter.
- Do not hang pacifiers on cords or ribbons around a child's neck. Use pacifiers with ventilation holes and a guard shield that is too large to fit inside the mouth.

Playground and Outdoor Safety

The U.S. Consumer Product Safety Commission reports that approximately 400,000 children are injured each year on the nation's playgrounds and that 25% of these injuries are treated in hospitals. An estimated 20 children die every year as a result of a playground injury.

Safety guidelines for playgrounds include:

- Be certain that there is sand, pea gravel, mulch, or a mat under all playground equipment.

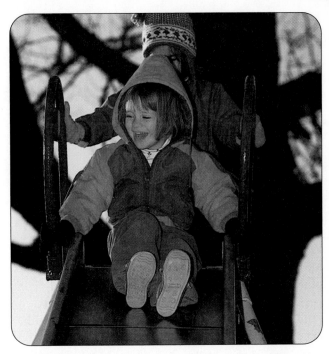

Figure 17-5 To ensure children's safety on the slide, only allow one child to slide down at a time.

- Use playgrounds where the swings are separate from the play area to reduce the chance of a child being struck by a swing.
- Swing seats should be sling-style and made from canvas or hard rubber. Avoid seats made of metal or wood to minimize an injury to a child struck by a swing seat. Sling-style seats also discourage children from trying to swing standing up.
- Use the bucket-style swings for toddlers.
- Proper slide safety includes: keeping one arm's length between children climbing up the stairs, climbing up the steps rather than up the slide, and letting only one child at a time slide feet first and immediately moving from the bottom of the slide (▲ **Figure 17-5**).
- During hot weather, check the temperature of a metal slide with your hand before you allow a child to slide down.
- Slides and climbing structures should be no higher than 6′ for children under age 8, with a maximum of 8′ for older children.
- Allow children on a seesaw only if the structure is affixed in sand, pea gravel, or pine bark mulch, and then only with supervision.
- Do not lift a child to reach a climbing structure. If it is too high for the child to reach, it is too advanced for the child's ability.
- Rake sandboxes regularly for debris. Cover a back yard sand box to keep animals out of it.

- Fence in your outdoor play area.
- Place plastic caps over protruding sharp ends and screws if you have a metal swing set.
- Inspect wooden climbing structures routinely, and sand rough areas to prevent splinters.
- Do not allow children to play behind parked cars in the driveway.

Bicycle Safety

Bicycle riding is good exercise and is enjoyed by people of all ages. However, bicycles are associated with a high number of accidents and injuries. The U.S. Consumer Product Safety Commission has issued safety regulations for bicycle manufacturers to eliminate or reduce the risks of injury associated with design, construction, and performance. Yet this solves only part of the problem. Adults, whether supervising child riders or cycling with child passengers, must always keep safety in mind.

Tricycle safety guidelines for younger children include:

- Have a tricycle available that fits the child today, not one to grow into later. A tricycle that is too large can be hard to control, and one that is too small can be unstable under a vigorous rider.
- Consider using the style of tricycle that has a seat low to the ground and at the same level as the pedals. This style is more stable than models with a high seat and low pedals.
- Allow only one child at a time to use a tricycle.
- Allow children to ride on flat surfaces only; be sure that motorists can see the child.
- Check tricycles for wear, sharp edges, and loose or missing parts. Store in a garage or under cover to prevent rust, which weakens metal.

Safety guidelines for riding a bicycle with a child passenger include:

- Passenger bicycle seats are recommended for use beginning at 1 year of age. When purchasing a bicycle seat, choose a model with a seat back that extends high enough to protect the child's head; the seat should also come with protective plastic that covers the bicycle spokes to prevent feet from getting caught in them. Do not use a bicycle seat if any of the parts are missing.
- Wear a helmet yourself and use a properly-fitted child helmet.
- Adjust the seat belt so that the closure is on the outside back of the seat instead of across the lap. That way, only you can unbuckle it.

- Remember that the child's additional weight will make pedaling more difficult and the bicycle less stable. Braking time is increased and downhill cruising speeds can increase without your noticing.
- Pick safe routes. Do not bike in wet weather, when visibility is reduced; tires can skid, and wet hand brakes do not work effectively.

Car Safety

Car accidents are, by far, the leading cause of injury and death to children from ages 1 to 14. Most children injured or killed in motor vehicle accidents are not restrained in car safety seats or seat belts. All 50 states, the District of Columbia, and Puerto Rico have child passenger safety laws making it illegal and punishable by a fine to transport a child in a vehicle who is not in a child safety seat, booster seat, or properly adjusted seat belt. Restrained children are less likely to distract the driver and more likely to nap or look at books and toys. A child who uses a safety seat beginning in infancy is not aware of any other way to travel and, as the child grows, is more likely to accept safety seats and seat belts as a way of life (**Figures 17-6, 17-7, and 17-8 ▶**).

All infants and children in safety seats and older children up to the age of 12 should ride in the back seat of the vehicle because it is the safest location. The center of the back seat ensures the greatest safety. Riding in cars equipped with front passenger air bags makes it even more critical to keep children in the back seat. Their small size makes them susceptible to serious head and neck injury and even death resulting from the impact of an inflating air bag if they are in the front seat during a collision.

Child safety seats come in a variety of sizes and styles. Choose one that is easy to use and fits properly in your car. Install it exactly as the manufacturer instructs and use it every time you get into the car. A car seat used part-time is risky. A car seat used improperly is as dangerous as no restraint at all. There are also specially-made car seats and car beds available for medically fragile children and premature infants. In some vehicles, a child passenger restraint system is built into the center back seat.

Did You Know?

In a 30-mph car accident, an unrestrained child hits the dashboard or windshield with the same force as if the child fell from a third-floor window.

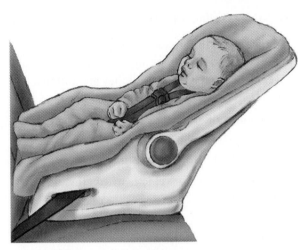

Figure 17-6 Infant car seat (infant faces seat).

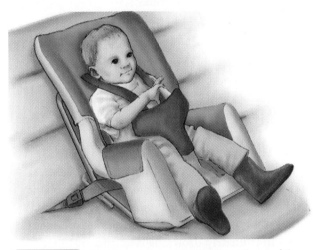

Figure 17-7 Toddler car seat (toddler faces front of the car).

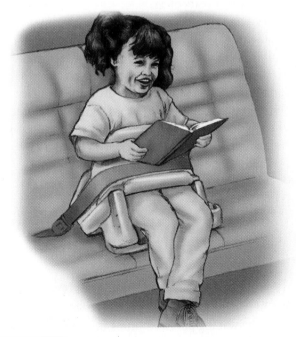

Figure 17-8 Booster seat.

Your responsibility checklist includes the following:

- Set an example for using seat belts with your positive attitude and your consistency in using them.

- Use a child safety seat or booster seat that meets or exceeds government safety standards. Secure seats only on the rear seat of the vehicle.

- Place infants up to one year old and weighing up to 20 pounds in an infant safety seat facing backwards. Place children weighing between 20 and 40 pounds in a safety seat facing forward.

- Place children weighing between 40 and 80 pounds in a belt-positioning booster seat. Children who are this size have outgrown safety seats but are not big or tall enough for the adult-sized restraint. A booster seat incorporates the adult lap belt and shoulder restraint. Some models have a padded shield in front of the child. The child should use the booster seat until large enough for the adult lap belt to rest across the pelvis, not the abdomen, and for the shoulder belt to be away from the neck and face. If the belt rests across the child's abdomen, it could result in a serious internal injury in a collision. Never tuck the shoulder restraint portion of an adult belt behind a child seated in a booster seat because this leaves the child vulnerable to injury.

- Never substitute a household booster seat or an infant play seat for a child safety seat.

- Do not allow children to share seat belts because the impact of a collision can crush one child against the other.

- Do not permit a child to ride on an adult's lap. An unrestrained child will be thrown from the adult's arms by the force of a crash. A child restrained on an adult's lap in the same belt will be crushed between the belt and the adult.

- Do not allow a child to sit on a driver's lap to pretend to drive or play with the controls.

- Always lock doors securely.

- Teach children to exit the car on the curb side and cross in front of the car, not behind it.

Did You Know?

The National Highway Traffic Safety Administration estimates that, with correct use, child safety seats could prevent 56,800 injuries and 519 fatalities per year.

- Never leave a child alone in a car.
- Remove the cigarette lighter.
- If the car has been in the sun in hot weather, touch the metal clasps of the child's car seat to check the temperature. Make sure that the child's skin does not touch hot metal.
- Keep a survival kit in the vehicle's trunk. It should include a blanket, flares, a flashlight, and batteries.

Pedestrian Safety

Short walks near home or to and from a playground provide opportunities to teach safe behavior on streets and sidewalks. Children should hold your hand or loops on a travel rope when walking in a group of children. A travel rope is made by tying plastic bracelets a few feet apart along a length of rope. Children are taught to always hold onto the bracelet while walking.

Child Passengers and Air Bags

The danger to children who come in contact with a deploying front seat air bag has led to recommendations that infants or children under age 12 never ride in the front seat of a car with a front passenger air bag. These air bags were designed to strike the chest of an average-size male. Children are particularly vulnerable to severe brain and spinal injuries from air bags, which deploy at the speed of approximately 200 mph and can strike them in the face. A number of infants and children have been killed by inflating air bags.

Many parents, however, are concerned about the safety of placing their infant in a rear-facing car seat in the back seat. The American Academy of Pediatrics stresses that a healthy infant buckled properly in a rear-facing car seat is safe. The risk of injury from riding in the front seat is greater than the chance the infant will need immediate attention while riding in the back.

Vehicles equipped with rear side-impact air bags pose an additional concern about the safety of child passengers. Children who are seated close to an inflating rear side-impact air bag are at risk for injury or death from the impact of the air bag. The National Highway Traffic Safety Administration suggests that car owners have their rear side-impact air bags deactivated by their dealer if young children will be riding in the car.

When walking outdoors, teach the following safety steps:

- Teach children to stop just before the curb or edge of the road and to wait for an adult. Children should never step into the street until they are told that it is safe to go.
- Talk about traffic, pedestrian lights, and signs so that the children learn to recognize them.
- Teach children that vehicles can injure them.
- Teach how to look for vehicles when crossing an intersection.
- Teach children that people stay on the sidewalks, and vehicles stay on the street.
- Teach children to stay away from parked vehicles on the street and in driveways.
- Teach children to cross in front of a car or bus, not behind it, when they exit from the vehicle.
- Remind older children, who may cross streets regularly, not to be distracted by conversation.

Water Safety

Children are attracted to water—whether it's in a swimming pool, wading pool, bath tub, or bucket. They are attracted to the light reflecting off a pool, they like the sound of the water running into the bathtub, and they want to get their hands in a bucket of water to splash. Unfortunately, drowning is second only to motor vehicle accidents in the number of accidental deaths to children under 5 years of age.

A drowning can occur in only a few inches of water. The household bathtub is a common location for infant drowning. Every year, several thousand children are treated in hospital emergency rooms or are admitted for long-term care because of near-drowning injuries. This ever-present concern for safety in and around the water should keep the supervising adult constantly alert to the children's activity. Reduce the risk of injury by following these guidelines:

- If you own a pool, learn CPR.
- Keep your eyes on children around water. Never leave them unsupervised in a bathtub or any size pool, no matter how shallow the water or how short the time.
- Make certain that an adult is always present when a wading pool or bathtub is being filled.
- Empty wading pools, bathtubs, and water buckets immediately after each use.

- Keep the toilet lid down.
- Arrange for a child to learn to swim at a young age. Teach the child respect for water.
- Keep rescue flotation devices near a pool.
- Use caution in allowing nonswimmers to use a flotation device, including kickboards, in deep water. Even a momentary loss of grip on the device can cause panic and lead to drowning.
- Remove a ladder from an above-ground pool when it is not in use.
- Make certain that gates around a pool are securely locked when it is not in use. If neighbors have pools, make certain that they know that you care for children and discuss your safety issues with them.
- Never leave a child alone near a frozen body of water.

Growing Up Safely

When children are very young, childproofing is essential. This means that adults must make the world safe for the curious and exploring child who is too young to understand dangers or to make safe choices. As children grow, they leave this carefully controlled environment and must be taught to safely negotiate all of the experiences at school, on the playground, at home, or in someone else's home when an adult might not be present.

As children grow, you must warn them of hazards that they might encounter. Share with them the following safety rules for older children as they begin to do more for themselves and are exposed to more choices.

Sports and at Play

- Learn how to swim. If swimming is not a favorite activity, learn how to tread water and float on your back for your own safety. Learn the drownproofing techniques that keep you afloat while conserving energy.

Did You Know?

Approximately 300 children drown each year in neighborhood pools.

Source: Center for Environmental Health and Injury Control, Centers for Disease Control.

- Never swim alone or in dangerous areas such as a quarry or near a dam. Swim only with a lifeguard present.
- Never dive into shallow water, because hitting the bottom forcefully can break the neck.
- Wear a life jacket when boating or water skiing.
- Never ice skate alone on a frozen pond.
- Never run into the street after a ball or pet.
- Do not play in construction areas, on railroad tracks, or in abandoned buildings.
- Use a trampoline only when an adult is present. Only one person jumps at a time.
- When in-line skating or skateboarding, wear a helmet, protective padding and wrist braces. Skate on smooth surfaces only.
- Never carry more than 10% of your total body weight in a back pack.

Bicycle Riding

- Ride a bicycle that suits your height. A bicycle that is too large makes steering and braking difficult ▼ Figure 17-9 .

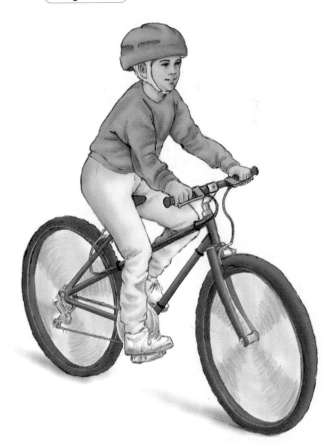

Figure 17-9 Wearing a helmet is a critical part of bicycle safety.

- Wear a helmet and clothing designed for biking. Keep shoes tied and wear leg bands on loose-fitting pants to reduce the risk of entangling clothes in the chain or sprocket.

- Do not ride a bike in bare feet.

- Equip the bicycle with reflectors.

- Do not hang onto a moving vehicle while on a bicycle, skateboard, in-line skates, or scooter.

- Do not give a ride to another person.

- Ride on bike paths. If you must use roads, travel in a single file on the right-hand side of the road. Use correct hand signals and obey all lights and signs for motorists. Watch for opening car doors and for cars pulling out of driveways and parking spaces.

- Avoid riding after dusk and in wet weather when visibility is reduced; tires skid, and wet handbrakes do not grip well.

- Do not clown around or perform stunts.

Bicycle Helmets Make Sense

+ Bicycle injuries are the most common cause of sports or recreational injury in the United States.*

+ Three of every four children who are hospitalized for a bicycle injury do not wear helmets even after they recover.**

+ The use of approved bicycle helmets reduces the risk of severe head injuries by 85%.***

+ 75% of all fatalities in bicycle-related accidents are the result of head injury.*

+ In a bicycle accident, you have a 50/50 chance of hitting your head.*

+ A fall from a bicycle that is moving at 20 mph will likely result in death if the rider's head hits the pavement, rocks, or another solid object.*

Sources:
*Injury Prevention Resource and Research Center, Dartmouth Medical School.
**National Head Injury Foundation.
***National Safety Council.

Electricity and Fire

- Never go near a downed or broken power line. The line might still be live and could kill anyone who gets too close to it. Never play near or climb on the fencing around an electric substation. Never climb an electric utility pole.

- Never touch an electrical appliance, even if it is turned off, if your hands or feet are wet because of the risk of electrocution. This also means you should not use a blow dryer or other electrical appliance while in the bathtub or shower.

- Never throw water on a plugged-in appliance on fire because of the risk of electrocution.

- Never stick anything other than an electrical plug into a wall outlet.

- Always hold the rubber grip when plugging or unplugging an electrical cord. Never touch the metal prongs. Never pull on the cord.

- Never fly a kite or hold onto a mylar balloon near a power line. Mylar balloons are safest indoors.

- Do not play with matches, lighters, or fireworks. Knowing that many children suffer burns from such activities should make the fun not worth the risk.

- If bread gets stuck in the toaster, do not try to get it out while the toaster is plugged in. Unplug the toaster before retrieving the toast.

- If food catches on fire in the microwave, turn off the microwave and leave the door closed; the fire will go out.

- Always tie back long hair when cooking over an open fire.

Personal Safety

- Do not walk toward a stranger who offers food or gifts or who asks for directions. Adults who need assistance should find another adult.

- When crossing a street, do not be distracted by conversation or by fooling around with friends.

- If walking at dusk or later, always wear white because it shows up well for drivers. If there is no sidewalk, walk on the left side of the road facing the traffic, and stay away from the edge of the road.

- At the first rumble of thunder, get out of water.

- If you become lost in the woods, find shelter and wait to be rescued. Moving from place to place increases the chance of being missed by adults searching for you.

- Never put your tongue against anything metal when outside during freezing weather because it will stick, and you will be injured if you try to pull it free. The same is true for things inside the freezer.

- Never put your fingers into the garbage disposal, even if it is not running.

- Never get into or put anyone inside a car trunk or old refrigerator because the person might suffocate.

- Never inhale the fumes of a chemical to "get high." It is extremely dangerous to your brain, liver, and nervous system.

- Ride only on the inside of a vehicle. Do not ride on the bumpers, hood, trunk, or other exterior surfaces.

- Until you reach the age of 13, ride only in the back seat of a vehicle because it is the safest seat. If the car has front seat airbags, you could be seriously injured by the airbag inflating in a collision.

- Always buckle your car seat belt, even if others in the car do not (Figure 17-10 ▶).

- Never, never get in a car if the driver has been drinking alcohol or using drugs.

Firearms Safety

It is estimated that almost half of American homes with children have one or more handguns. Homicides are a leading cause of injury-related death in children under the age of 18, followed by suicide. The National Center for Health Statistics reports that, every day in America, 16 children under the age of 20 are killed in gun homicides, suicides, and unintentional shootings, and many more are injured or wounded. Approximately 66% of all homicides and more than half of all suicides among children involve handguns. In addition, approximately 16% of all unintentional firearm deaths occur in children under the age of 18 who were "just fooling around when it went off."

The increased availability and use of handguns can only ensure that the number of children injured and killed by them will continue to rise. Children alone at home after school with access to firearms present an unknown potential for serious injury and death.

Children are curious by nature and the lure of the forbidden when a firearm is accessible creates the potential for a disaster. Few children under the age of 8 can reliably tell the difference between a real gun and a toy gun. The difference in weight between a real gun and a toy gun does not register as an important indicator of danger to a child. Children should play with only brightly-colored toy guns, so that they can clearly understand the difference between what is play and what can kill. Consider disposing of toy guns that look like real ones.

It is worthwhile finding out if firearms are present in the homes of relatives and friends, because approximately 40% of shootings that involve children occur in these homes. Most occur when children are not supervised. Pump air guns, air rifles, air pistols, and BB guns can also cause injuries and deaths. Projectiles from these weapons can reach speeds comparable to some handguns and can penetrate skin and bone. No firearm should ever be present in a child care center or in a house or apartment where home-based child care is provided.

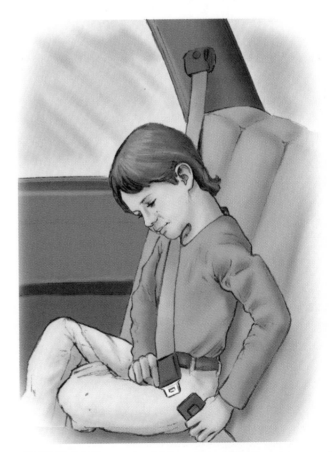

(**Figure 17-10**) Teach children about the importance of seat belts.

Learning Activities

Preventing Childhood Injury

Directions: Circle Yes if you agree with the statement, and circle No if you disagree.

Yes   No   **1.** Childhood injuries are often related to the child's level of development.

Yes   No   **2.** To avoid burn injuries, the temperature of a hot water heater should not exceed 150°F.

Yes   No   **3.** The warning signs of lead poisoning make it easy to recognize and treat.

Yes   No   **4.** Bicycle seats are recommended for use by children over the age of 6 months.

Yes   No   **5.** Allow 2 children to buckle into 1 car seat belt if there are not enough belts.

Quick Emergency Index